M000008566

DEDICATION

This book is dedicated to my Mom and Dad.

ACKNOWLEDGMENT

To all the people who patiently worked with me, let this be my chance to thank them.

DISCLAIMER

Be informed that this book is solely written based on my personal experience and I, in no way claim, that the information in it is 100% verified, as there is more and more research coming every day, discretion is advised. Furthermore, nothing contained herein is to be construed as Medical Advice. Use of any supplements/drugs and exercise regimen should only be done under the directions and auspices of a licensed physician. The writer does not claim to be a medical doctor, nor does he purport to issue medical advice.

CONTENT

1. Introduction   Pg#6
   a. AgileFitness and My Mission   Pg#8

2. Section 1: Fitness and Wellness Pillars   Pg#10
   a. The basics   Pg#11
   b. Mental and Emotional Fitness   Pg#13
   c. Rules for building internal motivation   Pg#15
   d. Purpose, passion and grit   Pg#16
   e. How to reduce stress   Pg#20
   f. How to build good habits   Pg#23
   g. Mental Fitness: creativity   Pg#25
   h. Meditation: why, what, how   Pg#27
   i. Breathing, Focus, yoga   Pg#29
   j. How to improve luck   Pg#30
   k. The true value of your time   Pg#33

3. Section 2: Training and Workouts   Pg#36
   a. Physical Fitness: How to get started   Pg#38
   b. Training and body types   Pg#40
   c. Training and Muscle fiber type   Pg#42
   d. Bodyweight vs free weights vs machine   Pg#45
   e. Cardio, Compound or Isolation, TUT   Pg#51
   f. HIIT vs Cardio   Pg#55
   g. Workout for beginners   Pg#56
   h. Top 10 common workout questions   Pg#58
   i. Good warm and recovery   Pg#62
   j. Your body set point and Benchmarks   Pg#66
   k. Soreness – good & bad pain   Pg#68
   l. Manual for 6 pack abs   Pg#72
   m. Increase agility and flexibility   Pg#77

n. How to create your own workout plan   Pg#82

o. Exercise for muscle building   Pg#86

p. Common Fat loss question   Pg#88

q. How to do spot fat reduction   Pg#91

r. How to double your plank hold time   Pg#97

s. How to increase biceps size quickly   Pg#98

t. Benefits of HIIT and Functional training   Pg#102

u. Workout for plus size overweight people   Pg#104

v. Exercise and menstrual cycle for women   Pg#105

w. Improve long distance running   Pg#108

x. Spiritual Fitness   Pg#110

y. Powerful morning routine for success   Pg#113

z. Discover your hidden happiness map   Pg#116

4. **Section 3: Nutrition and Weight Loss**   Pg#119

a. Measurement: BMR, Calories and lean mass   Pg#120

b. Healthy eating diet plans, recipes   Pg#124

c. How to make a diet chart by yourself   Pg#126

d. How to eat healthy   Pg#128

e. How to quite sugar addiction   Pg#130

f. Keto, low card and insulin   Pg#134

g. DIY- Protein bar and healthy snacks   Pg#138

h. Tips to buy milk   Pg#140

i. Nutrition label and emotional eating   Pg#142

j. What to eat before & after workouts   Pg#145

k. How to keep weight off throughout the years   Pg#149

l. Build lean muscle mass on Indian diet   Pg#151

m. How to Eat Out Without Getting Fat   Pg#152

n. Supplementation: Protein, Creatine, BCCA   Pg#154

o. How to convince your family to stay healthy   Pg#160

5. **Section 4: Longevity & Bio Hacks**   Pg#162

a. Longevity   Pg#163
b. Top 10 leading cause of death   Pg#163
c. Define your health KPIs   Pg#164
d. Essential habits to enhance longevity   Pg#168
e. How to stay young by 10 years   Pg#170
f. How to fix sleep issues naturally   Pg#172
g. How to stop common cold forever   Pg#173
h. How to recover fast from sickness   Pg#174
i. Rehab – heat, cold and stretching   Pg#177
j. How to have a highly productive day   Pg#179
k. How to stay in shape while travelling   Pg#184
l. The importance of the right breathing   Pg#185
m. Fitness for Professionals and Busy People   Pg#189

6. **Section 5: Future of Health and Fitness**   Pg#192
a. Healthcare and Fitness Integration   Pg#193
b. Artificial Intelligence (AI) and Healthcare   Pg#194
c. Sensors and e-health   Pg#196
d. Genome, Stem Cells, 3D Printing   Pg#200
e. The Future of Fitness   Pg#201
f. Top 10 health trends for 2020s   Pg#204
g. Role of Fitness trainer in Future   Pg#205
h. Five Eco hacks to reduce waste   Pg#208
i. Conclusion & Summary   Pg#211

7. **Reference**   Pg#212

INTRODUCTION

First of all, let me congratulate you. You wouldn't have taken time to start reading it if you were not ready to learn and change. This shows you're ready to begin exploring your fitness & health transformation journey.

Agile Fitness & My Mission

When I see people with poor health or physical condition, I understand that they lose a great opportunity to live a quality life. And when people tell me they don't have time to exercise, I don't think any less of them. I just think they don't know what they're missing.

I also understand that most of us are not celebrities who roam around with their personal chefs who cook us personalized high protein meals! We don't even have a lot of money to spend on all sorts of pre-workouts, fat-burners, hydro-whey, and all that high-end expensive stuff. So, there is none of those luxuries that glamour brings, you do not need any of that. We need to learn to do the best with whatever we have available in our time and budget.

I decided to write this book to share my experience and experiments-based learning knowledge around fitness, health, beauty and longevity. I am a Certified Fitness Trainer, Certified Nutrition Coach, Author and a Speaker. Most importantly I have spent the last one decade helping thousands of people and doing deep research and investigation about what it takes to not only get the body that you want, and the body that you deserve but also how to feel good, to look good and to perform as optimally as possible.

Mainstream health advice is often less than optimal, and in many cases completely ineffective and sometimes dangerous. Just a few years ago, after following popular health and fitness advice, I had chronic fatigue. Doctors could do nothing. I was getting sick frequently and I realized that life is not just about looking physically fit. Instead it is about complete optimization of your fitness, your health, your beauty in a long-term sustainable way.

My long journey through health led me to daily fitness and wellness practice, a whole unprocessed food diet, and to the science of physical fitness and anti-aging. I experimented with what is the minimum effective dose of exercise it takes to optimize in all these areas. And, what it takes to live a long healthy life that you want and feel as good as possible while living your life. Choosing the ideal state of Fitness, Health, Beauty and Longevity is not hard. You just need to know what to do. I have tried to systematize it for you in this book in short and easy to read sections.

This book doesn't aim to give you a workout or a diet plan. You can find any information and advice online about fitness, workout or healthy diet. This book is for giving you the easy to understand framework, actionable tips and bio hacks to feel what I call "AgileFitness"- Physically, Mentally, Spiritually and Emotionally Fit.

What is AgileFitness?

Agile Fitness is the name of my Fitness Venture. I choose this name because:

Life is dynamic and changing pretty fast. You do not know when your personal and professional life can throw a curveball against you. **Agile** means being able to adapt to changing situations easily and make tiny improvements on a consistent basis to transform your life.

Fitness means "readiness". Fit people are better equipped than non-fit people - physically, mentally, emotionally and socially.

What is my mission?

"My goal is to help at least ten million people to rediscover and redefine their health & fitness level, while having fun". If you want to achieve your goals and show others what your worth – the best way is to start to improve yourself.

You don't need to be perfect to inspire others. Let others get inspired by the way you deal with your imperfections. If you were able to believe in Santa Claus for ten years, believe yourself for at least one tenth as long and see the magic.

A Framework to transform yourself

I think the best way to change the world is to keep improving yourself in all areas of wellness and start helping the people you work with. Think about it this way: take any area of your life. Improve 1% a day at it. Just 1% compounded, that's 3800% a year. That's ENORMOUS improvement versus everyone else who is complacent or who does not know how to get 1% better. Just 1% a day, your life transforms and world changes.

As you will improve and have a good life then the world will also become a better place to live. You will start being more kind, honest, humble and will appreciate your life a lot more.

First, I wrote this book for myself to carry it with me during the day. I want to refer to learnings captured in this book whenever I have a question or need motivation. Then I shared it with a few friends, and they suggested that I publish this so it can help others as well.

The Book is NOT a fitness program, so you won't be subjected to long, grueling workouts or a strict diet plan. Instead, this book provides an easy-to-follow process to systematically enhance your overall wellness, so you develop a body that looks great, feels great, works at its full potential, and lasts.

I hope you will also find it helpful with lots of practical tips and tricks and can use it as your daily pocket fitness book on the go.

Note: Please read this book as a grain of Salt. And consult your doctor before doing any new workout or making any dietary changes.

SECTION 1

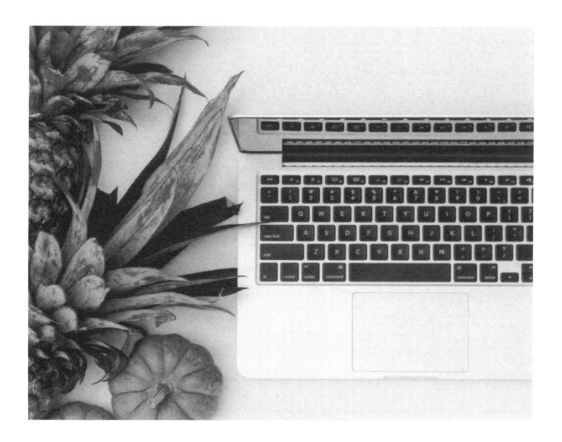

FITNESS AND

WELLNESS PILLARS

The Basics

Health is the new wealth. Health is the key to happiness. When you are sick in bed due to some chronic illness, it does not matter how much money you have in the bank.

Fitness and health should be seen as long-term and sustainable pursuits that can fit in your lifestyle. I see so many people get stuck in the endless loop of gaining weight and losing weight every year. Every year they have the same new year resolutions. They spend hours in the gym or doing some long form of endurance training but fail to apply the basics of health and wellness.

Let me be frank. You can get lean and ripped in one hour a week if you know how. Totally unnecessary to spend more time than that. But you need to build a good understanding of basics first. Let's dive into key pillars of fitness and wellness.

Key Pillars of Fitness and Wellness

I am a fan of having a good framework or mental model that you can use to bring changes and transformation in your life. Overall wellness and a good quality life are composed of many different areas. For simplicity, I have combined them into three key pillars. Our mind does a good job if we have to remember three things.

Another goal I had was to build this framework so that it's easy to follow whether you are in your 30s. 40s, 50, or even in your 80s.

There are 3 primary drivers of results in life:

1) Your luck (randomness).

2) Your strategy (choices).

3) Your actions (habits).

Only 2 of the 3 are under your control. But if you master those 2, you can improve the odds that luck will work for you rather than against you.

So, the question becomes how to make right choices and build the habits, the system, the relationships that can support you to achieve your designed fitness and quality of life that you want to live.

"When making plans, think big. When making progress, think small"

Best question to ask yourself at the beginning of year: every day, can I do 1% improvement in physical health, emotional health, creative health, and can I practice trying not to control the things I have no control over. Every single day.

We all should aim high to be great in 10 years. Build health habits today that lead to a great body in 10 years. Build social habits today that lead to great relationships in 10 years. Build learning habits today that lead to great knowledge in 10 years. Long-term thinking and compounded effects are a secret weapon.

Health is a state of being well. Here are four key pillars to health:
1. **Physical Fitness (Body)**
2. **Mental and Emotional Fitness (Mind)**
3. **Relationship & Spiritual Fitness (Heart and Soul)**
4. **Financial Fitness**

I am covering the first three pillars in this book. Financial health is a big enough topic of its own and I am still in process honing my financial fitness muscles.

Mental and Emotional Fitness (Mind)

We are all emotional human beings. Our emotion drives our behavior. Our behavior drives our habit. Our habits drivers who we become. Once you can put a word to your strengths, it becomes much more embedded in your everyday life".

One of my simple goals is that I want to be happy. Now happiness is a very loaded term. There are many different things that provide happiness to different people. For example, some people get happy by walking outside and others get happy after drinking alcohol. Let's understand what causes happiness and how to make good happiness choices.

Choose Your Happiness (Dopamine) Hits Wisely

Dopamine is a chemical produced by our brains that when released makes us feel pleasure. It's released in our brain whenever we get or expect to get a reward. So many different kinds of real-life rewards result in the release of dopamine: having a delicious meal, enjoying a glass of wine, the warm sand between our toes on a vacation, going on a long run, having sex, being praised by a colleague, a promotion at work, and so much more.

The pleasure associated with dopamine is strong and addictive and will ultimately motivate your actions, often unconsciously, to seek out more of the rewards in the hopes of ever more pleasure.

The challenge is that not all sources of dopamine are great for us. Drugs and alcohol, for example, are huge producers of dopamine, but can result in drug abuse and addiction that can trouble you for life.

Finding happiness is one of life's most important pursuits. I want more than anything for you to find your own happiness in whatever way makes sense for you. I've spent quite a bit of time reflecting on my own life and what has been crucial for creating a life full of it and I hope to share everything I've learned with you.

In the modern day there are a thousand of these little distractions, all promising small amounts of dopamine, that can ultimately leave us feeling needlessly anxious and unsatisfied. Yet even the small dopamine hits we get from these activities keep us coming back for more.

The way I think about dopamine is just like nutrition. There are various sources of dopamine just like there are various sources of calories. But it turns out the quality of those calories matter a lot. There are a lot of "empty calories" out there that we know are terrible for us: sugar, fast food, and more. So, we know we need to be mindful about where our calories come from.

The exact same thing is true for dopamine. I think it's entirely unrealistic to expect to live a life of non-attachment and avoid all sources of dopamine. But instead we should choose our dopamine hits wisely. We can pick which sources of dopamine we allow ourselves to indulge in just as we do the calories we choose to eat. And by doing so, guide our reward feedback loop to far superior sources of pleasure and ultimately happiness.

Every time we feel bored, anxious, angry, sad or lonely, we seek things that both numb the bad feeling and distract our attention with pleasure. One idea is to start dopamine fast by identifying the triggers and changing the environment.

Examples:

1) Put the stimulus (like your phone) away or make it harder to access.

2) Engage in an alternative activity that is incompatible with the stimulus (e.g. hard to do sports activity and stress eat at the same time)

3) Use website-blocking software or social accountability to prevent yourself from cheating.

OK. We now understand what makes us happy (for example: Sunbath, Yoga, Meditation, nature walk, reading book) and how to choose it wisely.

Next thing is how to have the ongoing motivation that can push you forward.

Four rules for building internal motivation

External motivation does not last. You read a motivational post or watch a video of someone. It provides you a temporary sense of motivation to do something. But it does not last. What you need is a system that can provide your ongoing internal motivation. Here are my three rules to build a lasting internal motivation.

1. **Purpose and Passion**
2. **Habits and Discipline**
3. **Perseverance/grit**
4. **After feeling**

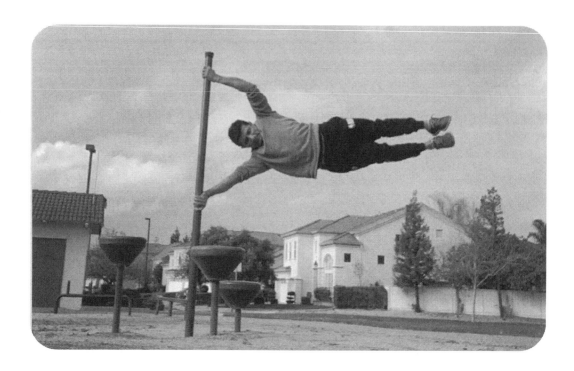

A simple example could be that pleasure after swimming/running/reading, realizing that will motivate you more and more. How you feel after doing an activity will attract you towards that good habit more and more.

Most people need consistency more than they need intensity.

Intensity: Run a marathon, write a book in 30 days, 10 days silent meditation retreat
Consistency: Don't miss a workout for two years, eat healthy items with every meal, daily silence.

"Intensity makes a good story. Consistency makes progress."

Purpose and Passion

We are continually thinking about how to do this, how to do that. But we don't give enough attention to what we are actually trying to accomplish, and why we are chasing it. If your "What" and "Why" are not clear, the "How's" will take you nowhere.

Purpose

Your purpose is not just your goal. For example, I want to be fit enough to run again. But it also includes your why – "so I can get back to playing my favorite sport.".

If you've decided now's the time to get fit and healthy, consider what made you realize this. Do you really miss something fun and active you used to do? Have you always wanted a muscular physique? Maybe, like me, you want to set a good example for your kids. That 'why' will help you power through when you are feeling low and do not want to get out of your cozy bed at 5am in the morning.

Once you've got your why, set yourself a goal. By setting an achievable goal with a clear timeline, you're setting yourself up for success.

Passion

If you could do one thing to transform your life, I would highly recommend it be to find something you're passionate about and do it for a living.

One of the most common stumbling blocks to launching a passion-based life is figuring out what you're passionate about in the first place. Experiment every day. Find out what sticks and see if it brings euphoria to your life while doing it.

Here are some techniques to discover your passion area. Now, this isn't as easy as it sounds, but it's well worth the effort.

Think about:

- The things you can do for your whole life without getting paid.
- The things that you talk to everybody and talk for hours.
- The things that you learn quickly.
- The places where you can spend hours without getting bored.
- The work that you do not think about retirement.
- What moves you... your energy never drains out.
- Things that make you curious.
- Things that bring joy, money, movement & progress.
- Anything that you loved to do in childhood.

Once you find out what you are passionate about go with full flow and force. Passion will provide you a growth lever if you can stick with it for some period of time. Find the growth lever and crank them to maximize the results.

Discipline

Ninety Percent of life is about showing up on time. To take advantage of our total potential, we need to be on time. Compounding impact takes care of overall progress over a period of time.

When starting a new training regime, be realistic. If you have been inactive for some time, know that the first week is going to be a struggle – but that every little bit of movement helps. If you're at the gym and see someone crushing an exercise you can't do, know that it will take time and practice and that everyone's journey is different.

If in these moments you find yourself thinking about giving up, put that discipline into action.

I want people to understand that you can do it. Getting comfortable with being uncomfortable is what it's all about. That's the hardest part of life – when we get uncomfortable, we tend to quit, or we tend to move away. And sometimes greatness is right beyond that. If you can just push through, that greatness is right there.

Every action you take is a vote for the type of person you wish to become. No single instance will transform your beliefs, but as the votes build up, so does the evidence of your identity. This is why habits are crucial. They cast repeated votes for being a type of person that you are or could become.

Perseverance and grit

These are about applying that discipline over time, over and over and over again 'till you reach your goal.

If you fall down, get back up. If you can't do it, practice and try again. If the road to your goal seems long, take it one step at a time.

The only thing to focus on in the beginning is to put in your reps. Your 1st workout will be weak, but your 1000th will be strong. Your 1st meditation will be scattered, but your 1000th will be focused.

A goal, especially if it's a big change from where you're currently at, can seem intimidating. So, break your long-term goal into smaller steps or mini goals. For example, training for five minutes longer than you did last week or make it through a full workout without taking extra breaks.

When you die, the sun will rise, the ocean will flow, all will go on with their life. As if you never existed. So, do what you really want to do. And don't forget, when it comes to achieving peak performance, a strong mind will help you combat physical and mental stress and keep on keeping on.

It will be a rocky road when you are trying to transform your mind, body and life. Some of the bad old habits and comfort zones will block you from making fast progress. The stress will build up. So, another basic life skill we need to learn is how to avoid constant stress in the modern world.

How to reduce stress (cortisol)

Cortisol is the stress hormone. More cortisol means:

- Harder to lose fat.
- Easier to lose muscle.
- FAR more likely to develop other health problems.

No joke - cortisol is one of the biggest causes of long-term health problems in our modern culture. Continuously elevated levels of cortisol can slowly destroy your delicate adrenal glands and disrupt your health and physiology. Having intermittent stress is not a problem, but if you remain under stress for weeks without recovering from it then it can bring many problems. Stress will come from many different angles. Stress on your body, stress on your mind and stress is on your soul.

I've found eight most practical and effective ways to conquer the stress which can fit for almost anyone.

Sleep. Number one is sleep, and for a reason. One of the biggest reasons people never really experience drop-in stress levels, is due to lack of sleep. Sleeping only 4-6 hrs. isn't enough. Stress is usually an accumulation. And sleep prevents this build up

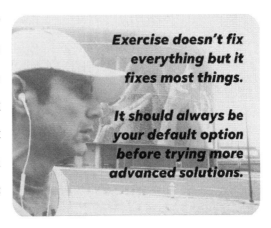

Exercise doesn't fix everything but it fixes most things.

It should always be your default option before trying more advanced solutions.

Exercise. Full Body Training. This means:
1. Shorter workouts (45 mins or so)
2. 3 days off (as recovery days) per week.
3. If your workouts are well over 1 hour, your stress will rise. If you don't have enough days off, your stress levels will rise.

Eat Nutritious Foods. Choo   se less processed food, cut down on sugar and seed oil.

Meditation (any type that can keep you calm for 12-15 minutes). Meditating has proven time and time again to reduce stress levels. If you currently struggle to sleep, then I recommend doing this just before bed for best results. Breathing (slow box breathing) is a great way to start if you are sort on time. It's time we learn to sit alone with our thoughts.

Maintain Good Relationships. Spend time with a loved one. Maintain good relationships, and you'll keep cortisol down, and testosterone up.

Do hobby/fun activity. Finding out what you enjoy doing is important. Fun is also a requirement - just make sure it DOESN'T include boozy weekends! Walk in Nature. Listen to music. Try walking while listening to your thoughts to learn something about yourself. Walking with podcasts, music is good but does not help if you want to learn about yourself.

Reading. Another great hobby is Reading. Reading is like a software update for your brain. Whenever you learn a new concept or idea, the software improves. You download new features and fix old bugs. In this way, reading a good book can give you a new way to view your life experiences. Your past is fixed, but your interpretation of it can change depending on the software you use to analyze it.

Practice gratitude. You will have enough, and you will never have enough. Start appreciating what you have first. Otherwise life is a never-ending chase.

Get Enough Water. Most people need 2-4 liters per day, yet most get less than two. It's a very fast way to ensure that you maintain chronically high stress levels, especially when coupled with lack of sleep. Get enough water. Water mantra to stay healthy:

- Drink 1-liter water as soon as you wake up.
- Drink one small glass of warm water before going to bed.
- Always drink water while sitting
- Get into the habit of drinking warm water 45 mins after every meal
- Drink a glass of water 30 mins before taking shower

Another thing to note is that depression is rarely due to medical conditions (of course there are exceptions). The human body never goes "ill" without a REASON. People make themselves ill and depressed by
- Malnourished diet
- No Movement.

- Vegetable oils & sugar
- Drugs, Alcohol addiction
- Poor gut health
- No sunlight
- Victim mindset. You have the power to be in control of your health

How to Break a Bad Habit and Replace it with a Good One?

Most of your bad habits are caused by two things: Stress and boredom. Recognizing the causes of your bad habits is crucial to overcoming them

Most of the time, bad habits are simply a way of dealing with stress and boredom. Everything from biting your nails to overspending on a shopping spree to drinking every weekend to wasting time on the internet can be a simple response to stress and boredom.

But it doesn't have to be that way. You can teach yourself new and healthy ways to deal with stress and boredom, which you can then substitute in place of your bad habits.

You don't eliminate a bad habit, you replace it. Bad habits address certain needs in your life. And for that reason, it's better to replace your bad habits with a healthier behavior that addresses that same need. If you expect yourself to simply cut out bad habits without replacing them, then you'll have certain needs that will be unmet and it's going to be hard to stick to a routine of "just don't do it" for very long.

For example, if you smoke when you get stressed, then it's a bad plan to "just stop smoking" when that happens. Instead, you should come up with a different way to deal with stress and insert that new behavior instead of having a cigarette.

How to break a bad habit:

- Choose a substitute for your bad habit
- Cut out as many triggers as possible
- Join forces with family, friends.
- Surround yourself with people who live the way you want to live.
- Build your new identity. Visualize yourself succeeding

Whenever you want to change your behavior, ask yourself

1. How can I make it obvious?

2. How can I make it attractive?

3. How can I make it easy?

4. How can I make it satisfy?

Here's a simple way to start just track how many times per day your bad habit happens. Put a piece of paper in your pocket and a pen. Each time your bad habit happens, mark it down on your paper. At the end of the day, count up all of the tally marks and see what your total is. Breaking bad habits takes time and effort, but mostly it takes perseverance.

Example: Break Alcohol habit:

People say they drink because of these two reasons:

1. The pressure from the drinking group.

2. Drinking relieves stress.

Most people are pressured by others to drink alcohol or consume drugs. In fact, most people who would rather give up alcohol continue to drink it simply because everyone else does and they do not want to be funny in front of all the group just because he decided to never drink.

Here's a handy guide to navigating the first few months of your alcohol-free life – without alienating your friends.

- Let everybody know that you have stopped drinking. Mention it on your Facebook and Instagram.
- Nobody actually cares that you're not drinking. You're overthinking it if you think that they do.
- Make jokes about not drinking and show them that you don't care. People can't make fun of you if you have a light-hearted attitude about it
- Use excuses if you feel you must. There is no end to potential excuses you can make.
- Do not lecture others why they should not drink

Remember, you've made a choice. It's a sensible, healthy choice: more money, fewer empty calories or drunk-food choices, and without hangovers you'll have more time and motivation to hit the gym. Real friends will respect and appreciate that these things are important to you.

MENTAL FITNESS

Mental fitness involves creativity, mental toughness, clear thinking. These mental muscles are what separate someone from becoming great at whatever they do.

Build a Growth Mindset

If you start out with $100 at the beginning of the year and you are able to increase what you have by 1% every single day, at the end of the year, you will have $3,778.34 = $100 * (1 + 1%) ^ 365. That is 37.78x what you had at the beginning of the year. Wake up every day and ask yourself not only what the

1% improvement is I can change to make my professional and personal life better. Get that 1% every single day!

Creativity: Start training your Idea muscle

Every day I start writing down 10 ideas. Next day, if there's some itch from the list before you want to scratch, then write "10 ideas to execute on that one idea". DON'T FORGET: Execution ideas are just a subset of IDEAS. Make execution ideas easy so you can experiment.

The future is too complex and far away to worry about. Experiment/Do every day to find what you love. Then get 1% better each day. Experiment every day!

One great tool that falls under mental fitness is meditation. Let's understand why, what and how of meditation.

The creativity process is the act of making new connections between old ideas. Thus, we can say creative thinking is the task of recognizing relationships between concepts.

One way to approach creative challenges is by following the five-step process of 1) gathering material, 2) intensely working over the material in your mind, 3) stepping away from the problem, 4) allowing the idea to come back to you naturally, and 5) testing your idea in the real world and adjusting it based on feedback.

Being creative isn't about being the first (or only) person to think of an idea. More often, creativity is about connecting ideas. Start writing 10 ideas every day to improve your idea muscle.

Meditation: How to get started

When I started to explore meditation a few years ago, I had a big anxiety over whether I am going it right or not. After every session I used to think I could have done better. Another big problem I see is that people are not able to fit meditation in their current schedule or they do not enjoy their sessions.

Just think that everything in our lives is thought. There is no past and future. If we don't think about the past it disappears. If we don't think about the future it vanishes. There is only now, the present moment.

> *"Meditation is an exercise that trains your mind to regulate itself. It's the ability to focus on one thing continuously without a break".*

How to get a meditation habit?

The most popular activities for getting meditation habit are:

- ▢ Counting your breath: this practice is great for beginners.
- ▢ Guided meditation: following the instructions of a teacher in person or via an app/recording. Instructors will take you through various awareness exercises like counting your breath, scanning your body, noticing sounds and visuals around you. This is also very effective for beginners.
- ▢ Mindfulness Meditation: this is defined by expert Jon Kabat-Zinn as 'moment to moment non-judgmental awareness.' Related styles are Vipassana and Buddhist.

If you do the right meditation you will gain more energy throughout the day and will improve your brain work too.

For starting meditation, you will need: A place to sit, and A timer.

While sitting you should keep your back straight. You can either close or open your eyes. In a word, just choose a position that is more comfortable for you.

Tips to build a meditation practice:

- o Meditate every day. Block time on the calendar.
- o Start small- 2-5 minutes a day.
- o Try to meditate at the same time every day.
- o Meditate in a silent place.
- o Try counting for concentration.
- o Remember it is no good or bad.

Breathing & Yoga to Build Your Balance, Focus and Calmness

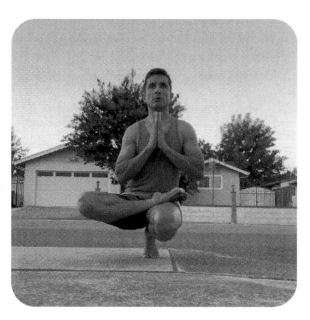

Breath control helps to be more focused increasing your concentration & performance.

Our breathing is controlled by the respiratory center of the brain. Our breathing rate and pattern changes when we are stressed which leads to more frustration and health problems.

Breath practicing starts with breath focus. Try to breathe slow and deep and remove all bad thoughts and worries. It will be more helpful if you can hold breath in your stomach.

Focus and concentration:

People that practice self-care have better cognitive ability, focus, and concentration.

Our mind consists of two parts. One helps us to focus and get things done, accomplish our ideas and get miracles in our career. But, unfortunately, the other one pulls us back. So, which one we will concentrate and allow to manage our life, will determine our success and the future. And this is because we are completely controlled by our minds.

Rules that will help you to develop focus

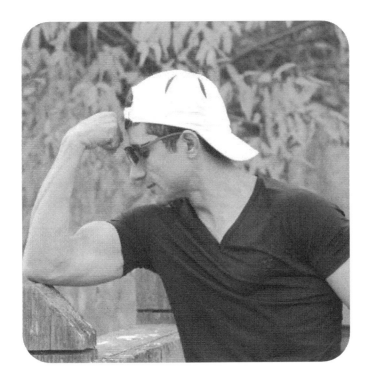

In order to engage in deep work, Newport says you need to develop a few habits:

1. Block out time. Schedule time on your calendar to work on something.

2. Create a focus and ignore list

3. Embrace boredom. Stay away from social media for a few hours.

4. Productive meditation.

5. Adopt a zero-tolerance policy.

6. Prepare for deep work and know the outcome.

7. The '20 percent less rule

List everything that you are trying to achieve, everything that makes you happy and is very important to you. Design your time around those things. Because time is your one limited resource and no matter how hard you try you can't work 24/7.

If you want to use your time wisely, you have to ask the equally important but often avoided complementary questions:

1. What don't you want to achieve?
2. What doesn't make you happy?
3. What's not important to you?
4. What stays in your way of achieving your goals?

The Law of attraction

Apparently, our mind continuously radiates waves in the universe. Our thoughts and beliefs also vibrate at certain frequencies and energy levels. If we desire something very strongly, the mind will send positive waves in the universe and will make circumstances to make the thing you want to happen (Quantum physics).

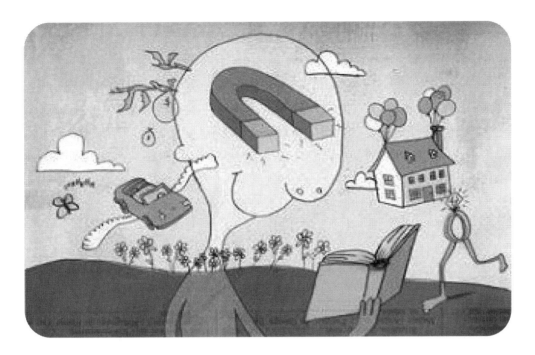

Now, if I try to connect the dots in mind and relate LOA to God and worship then it will make even more sense. There is a technique to keep you focused on your desires and get them quickly. You should visualize your desires and feel like they already came true. Focus on the benefits whether they are personal, materialistic, affecting others, achieving goals or other desires.

How to improve your luck?

"LUCK" is perhaps the most commonly used word in our day.

We often blame luck when bad things happen in our life, and we also call it luck when one gets or does something that we have never expected.

Perhaps, one can explain it as the invisible force behind the unexplained situations.

We have both bad and good things happening in our lives. No one is completely lucky in all his life. We rarely meet someone who says that he is

31

always lucky. But we all know at least a person who convinces that he is unlucky all the time. So, what is luck and what is it all about?

I think that everyone can sometimes be happy and sometimes be unhappy. It is all about our attitude and the way we see luck and the situation. Optimists always compare bad things that happen to them with worse that could have happened and feel lucky about it. Pessimists look at the bad that happened, compare it to the good that could have been and feel unlucky. Indeed, who is happier?

For me, perspective is the magic word. If you don't feel happy about something, just change the perspective. Look at the broader perspective, be optimistic and you will find all the happiness you ever wanted. That's what I call being lucky.

In other words, no one is born lucky or unlucky or even have good or bad times. Luck is not an external force; it is the inner feeling of a person. You can be facing the worst time of your life, being called so unfortunate by everyone around you, but still feel happy and lucky by changing your perspective.

Though I am not yet the happiest person in the world, but I am happy for whatever happens or is happening in my life.

Always tell yourself: "I am getting better than before"!

The REAL Value of Your Time

Time is our scarcest resource. Other resources like money and people can fluctuate up and down, but time only moves in one direction.

When I share this quote with others, they appear to get it — but then their actions prove otherwise. Most people still value money more than time and make decisions based on the present value of money vs. the future value of their money investment (ROI).

How to value your time

First, you need to value your time correctly.

Define your hourly rate. Let's assume you could make $75/hour ($150K/year) working a job. Determining your ROI now becomes straightforward: If you can hire someone or something to get a job done for less than $75/hour, you should.

At any given point in time, there are only a few key actions that matter. You need to put all your energy towards those actions and ignore the rest. The ROI calculation breaks down for certain intangibles that are way more valuable than money. We have solely been focusing on how to value time for work. But there are 3 more buckets that are just as critical to living a meaningful life:

Health	**Wealth**
Relationships	**Work**

Health

If you work harder than what is healthy, your health eventually suffers, and you may not be able to reap your eventual rewards at your fullest.

Relationships

If you work at the expense of your relationships, you may not have anyone with whom to enjoy your eventual rewards.

Wealth

You are investor #1 in your idea and need to be even more ruthless with its viability than your investors. They invest money. You invest time. Time is more valuable than money.

But despite your best efforts, startups are inherently uncertain, and you may still not have an eventual payoff. You need a plan B.

Consider this, putting aside just $300/month in the S&P 500 index fund would grow to ~$1M in 40 years. The ROI of automating something like this in your twenties (or thirties or forties) is crazy.

Work

And finally, doing good/original work comes from creativity. And recent studies show that creativity happens in the empty spaces between stretches of hard, focused work. In other words, you need to bake in free time for "doing nothing" in order to create something meaningful.

The way I balance these quadrants is with a calendar. Like most entrepreneurs, I am naturally driven to allocate most of my time to work. So, I first block off non-negotiable time on my calendar for the other 3 quadrants. Then prioritize my remaining time for work activities.

"What separates us is what we do with the 24 hours we are given every day. Don't waste it".

Within these key actions, you'll often find a mix of core jobs and non-core jobs.

Non-core jobs, like accounting, appointment scheduling can and should be delegated to less expensive services or tools. There is zero ROI in you doing these yourself.

Within core jobs, you'll find jobs you're good at, i.e. they fall within your personal superpowers, and jobs you're not yet good at. Trying to learn these skills on your own seems smart, but it isn't. A better approach is hiring a learning accelerator, like a book, or a workshop, or an expert — often in that order.

You are on time. Start today.

"New York is 3 hours ahead of California, but it does not make California slow.

Someone graduated at the age of 22 but waited 5 years before securing a good job! Someone became a CEO at 25 and died at 50. While another became a CEO at 50 and lived to 90 years.

Someone is still single, while someone else got married. Obama retires at 55, but Trump starts at 70.

People around you might seem to go ahead of you, some might seem to be behind you. But everyone is running their own race, in their own time. Don't envy them or mock them. They are in their TIME ZONE, and you are in yours!

So, relax. You're not late. You're not EARLY. You are very much ON TIME. Start now make today your day!

At any given point in time, there are only a few key actions that matter. We need to put all your energy towards those actions and ignore the rest.

SECTION 2

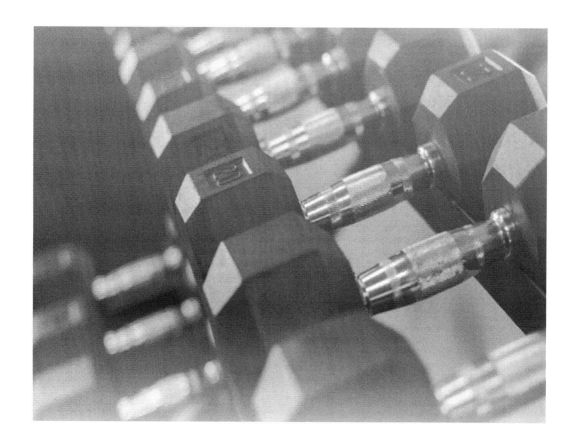

PHYSICAL FITNESS:

TRAINING AND WORKOUTS

PHYSICAL FITNESS

Motivation itself is merely an emotion. It is impossible to be happy or sad or angry 24 hours a day, and, it is also impossible to be motivated all the time. But when you feel that motivation, work on building a good healthy lifestyle habit. Do it before the motivation dies out. Remember, fitness is your right, but you have to earn it.

How to get started and build an exercise habit?

If your intention is to compete with the top specialists in your chosen career, sport or another discipline, then you should start by reforming and refining daily habits. Only then you can meet the criteria of excellence over time.

The great fitness people do what they have to do whether they feel like doing it or not. One day you will wake up and there won't be any more time to do the things you always wanted. Do it now.

Have patience when you have nothing and a good attitude when you have everything. Ambition is the first step. Fall in love with the process and the result will come.

Tips for building an exercise habit

1. Start exercising every day, not 2 or 3 times a week. You will be more consistent and will soon build a good habit of exercising every day. If you can exercise 21 days, then consider that you already have a habit and did the first step for a healthy life.
2. Set exact time for exercising and send reminders to yourself.

3. Though you should exercise every day, start small. Take small steps every day. Consider 10-15 minutes a day. If you do much at the beginning, you are likely to quit your habit very soon.

4. When your body will be ready to do more, then you can add your exercises. You can progress and exercise 20 minutes a day, and then day by day add the time to 50 minutes a day.

5. Have fun. Try to make the exercises easy and pleasurable for you.

6. Create a pleasant and right environment for the exercises. Choose the place where you feel comfortable and focus on the process, not the results. Don't forget, always have your purpose in your mind.

Example, how to make running fun?

Our Body is an adaptive BIO machine. For example, when you are running, your breathing stabilizes, your body develops muscle memory and it becomes easier to flow with every run. As you practice more, it gets easier and after a few months running becomes a natural activity for you.

But this means that your body is in its comfort zone. So, you will not progress any further. That's how most runners hit a plateau. Running the same distance at the same pace every day might be enjoyable but eventually, it stops pushing your body to change.

You have to change and do it differently every day if you want to get most out of your run. For example, you can run different distances, under different conditions, at different speeds, throw in some bodyweight and strength training sessions. That's how you keep your body sharp and force it to continue changing. Burn more every time and improve your speed, endurance, flexibility and overall fitness.

Here are some ideas that you can mix

- Endurance training: see just how far your body can take you at your lowest speed.
- Speed Drills: sprinting is the best way to push your body to the next level and gain momentum. Do at least one set of speed drills per week and watch how your body changes.
- Endurance & Speed: this is how you level up, first you push your body to endure long distance and then you force it into the final home run to sprint. Make it a 9 to 1 ratio. If you are running 10 kilometers, then your last 1-2 kilometers should be done at your top speed.
- Uphill: running is supposed to be challenging, finish your runs by running up a small hill and, if you run on a treadmill, change your incline level and go up. Try it at least once a week.
- Add Bodyweight workouts: Add some pushup & Squat to break the pattern and hyper load your muscle. Do jump squats, jump knee tuck exercises and skipping and straight leg bound drills in between your runs to improve your acceleration and speed.
- Extra weight runs - get a pair of wrist weights and run wearing them. Next day you will feel so light when running without the weight and go with increased speed.
- The more variety you have in your running the better results you'll get. You will perform better and you'll look better, too.

TRAINING AND WORKOUTS

If I were to get a dollar every time someone asked whether they should go for heavy weight, less rep or light weight, more reps, I'd probably be a millionaire.

A lot of people have this question and it's a genuine question too. Unfortunately, there is no one direct answer. I am going to explain how it all works and then maybe you can figure out what would work better for you. I'll also tell you my personal training regime and how it was better than others.

There are a lot of factors that matter when it comes to building muscles or losing fat, ranging from body type to genetics and what not. Different types of sports would require you to have different bodies, however since we're into building muscles and losing fat, I'll only discuss training which will be relevant to that.

Starting with body type, we have three major classifications:

1. ECTOMORPH

An ectomorph is the typical skinny guy. Ectomorphs have a light build with small joints and lean muscle. Usually ectomorphs have long thin limbs with stringy muscles. Shoulders tend to be thin with little width.

2. MESOMORPH

A mesomorph has a large bone structure, large muscles and a naturally athletic physique. Mesomorphs are the best body type for bodybuilding. They find it quite easy to gain and lose weight. They are naturally strong which makes for the perfect platform to build muscle.

3. ENDOMORPH

The endomorph body type is solid and generally soft. Endomorphs gain fat very easily. Endomorphs are usually of a shorter build with thick arms and legs. Muscles are strong, especially the upper legs. Endomorphs find they are naturally strong in leg exercises like the squat.

Now don't be disheartened if you are an ectomorph or endomorph, I am an endomorph, just saying! You must be thinking, "yeah so there is endo, etc., blah blah, who cares, where's my workout routine?" Well, hold your thoughts, we are getting there. It is important to understand a few things before you go there.

Since your primary goal is to build (or maintain) muscles, you need to understand them first. The following chart shows an overview of different types of muscles in the body:

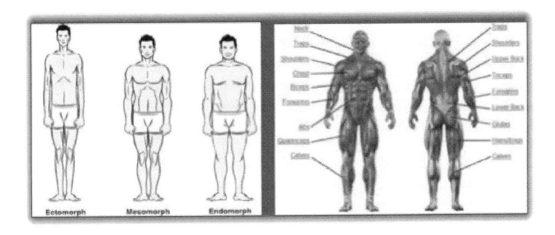

Your muscles are not all the same size and may require different types of stimulus to get stronger and developed. You cannot keep doing squats and expect to get a good chest. I know that is obvious and it is not what I am trying to say. What I mean to say is that the weight, the repetitions, the intensity and the form, all these are the factors that play an important part in giving the proper stimulus to any muscle group. So, if you were going to ask should I lift heavy weight and do less reps or lift lightweight and do more reps, it becomes clear as you read the next sections. There is no single answer, and no one size fits all here. Different athletes in the history of bodybuilding have shown and proved that you can build a great body by following different methods.

Muscle Fiber Types

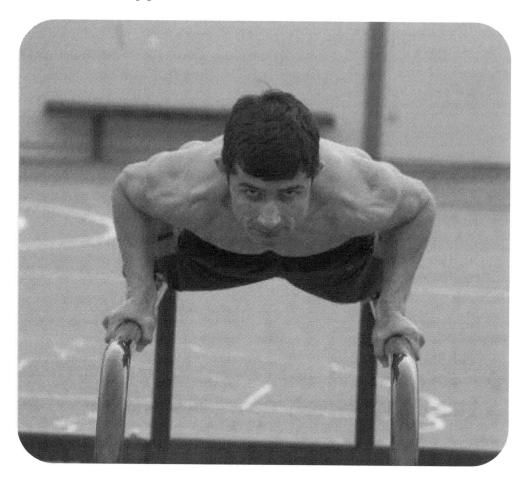

Though muscles are muscles, their composition can vary. It can have different proportions of two different kinds of muscle fibers: slow twitch and fast twitch.

So, your body has bundles of muscle fibers, and these bundles have varying proportions of these two types of fibers.

1. SLOW TWITCH

These are also known as Type 1 or red muscle fibers. They are responsible for long-duration, low intensity activity such as walking or any other aerobic activity.

2. FAST TWITCH

These are known as Type 2 or white muscle fibers (divided further into A and B). They are responsible for short-duration, high intensity activity.

Type 2B fibers are built for explosive, very short-duration activity such as Olympic lifts. Type 2A fibers are designed for short-to moderate duration, moderate-to-high intensity work, as is seen in most weight training activities.

By looking at elite athletes in different sports, you can see extreme examples of each make-up of muscle fiber. At the slow twitch end is the endurance athlete, such as the marathon runner.

These athletes can have up to 80% or more of slow twitch muscle fibers in their bodies, making them extremely efficient over long distances. At the fast twitch end is the sprinter. World-class sprinters can have up to 80% or more of fast twitch muscle fibers in their body, making them extremely fast, strong and powerful but with limited endurance.

How to Train Your Muscle Fiber Type?

When you're training with weights, your goal is to work as many muscle fibers as possible. Targeting more muscle fibers means greater gains in strength and muscle mass.

If your fibers in a particular muscle consist primarily of slow twitch fibers, in order to affect the greatest number of those muscle fibers, you'll need to train that muscle with higher reps, shorter rest periods and higher volume. This is because they take longer to fatigue, they recover quickly, and they require more work to maximize growth.

Unfortunately, slow twitch muscle fibers are limited in their potential for growth so even if a muscle group is primarily slow twitch, you should definitely include some

lower rep training to maximize the fast twitch fibers you've got in that muscle.

If you find you have a hard time gaining size in a particular muscle, it could be because it has a predominance of slow twitch muscle fibers. Higher reps (e.g. 12 to 15 reps), higher volume (more sets) and shorter rest periods (30 seconds to a minute between sets) can help you to maximize those muscles.

This doesn't mean you should use light weight, though. You should still strive to use weights that are as heavy as possible that will cause you to reach failure in those higher rep ranges. If you don't use heavy weights, you won't give your muscles a reason to grow.

If your fibers in a particular muscle group consist primarily of fast twitch muscle fibers, you're one of the lucky ones. Fast twitch muscle fibers have greater potential for size than slow twitch. The faster twitch fibers you've got, the greater your ultimate muscle size can be. These muscles are most likely the strongest and quickest to develop.

To maximize your muscles with fast twitch fibers, you'll need to train with low to moderate reps (e.g. 4 to 8 reps), rest period so far around 1 to 2 minutes and a moderate training volume (too much volume will compromise recovery).

If your muscles have a fairly even mix of fibers, you can evenly divide your training between focusing on the lower-rep, fast twitch fiber training and the higher-rep, and slow twitch fiber training. This will help you to develop all the fibers in your muscles, maximizing your ultimate development.

Bodyweight vs Free Weights vs Machines?

Which is better?

Resistance training or strength training: is there anything it can't do? From pumping up muscles to improving functional fitness and even igniting calorie burn for weight loss, resistance moves have serious benefits. Strength training is the ultimate life hack. It blows my mind so many people still don't do any. Here are some know benefits:

- Stronger for everyday tasks
- Less chance of injury
- Increased longevity
- Look better naked
- Improved posture
- More confidence
- Better health. It's a no brainer

But there are still some major misunderstandings about which style is best for different results. In the most basic and obvious sense, weight training exercises can fall into three different groups based on how they are performed and what type of equipment is used.

They are:

1. Free Weights

2. Body Weight Exercises
3. Machines

Despite what anyone else tells you, each type of exercise can serve a useful purpose in literally every workout routine regardless of what your goal is. However, certain types of exercises are definitely more ideal for certain people based on factors like experience level, training preferences, body type, genetics, and of course, your specific fitness goal.

So, let's go through how they compare with each other and what are their pros and cons. You'll then be able to easily determine which is best (and worst) for you.

1. Free Weights

A free weight exercise is any exercise where the resistance is provided by a barbell, dumbbells, or any other free moving object. Some common examples include any type of barbell or dumbbell press, row, curl, extension, or deadlift.

Basically, if you're moving some sort of weight (like a barbell or dumbbell) from point A to point B, and that weight isn't supported by or attached to anything other than you, it's most likely a free weight exercise.

Pros

1. Completely natural movement. Allows you to move through a range of motion that is completely natural for your specific body. Nothing is restricted or put into any sort of fixed position that may not be perfect for your body.
2. Uses additional muscles. Since you are in full control of the weight and stabilizing the entire movement itself, you are therefore recruiting the use of various stabilizer muscles that tend to go unused with machines.

3. Extremely functional. Free weight exercises allow you to mimic actual movements that you actually do in real life, and in the exact manner you'd actually do them.

4. Ideal for home use. If you happen to do your weight training at home, a barbell (or dumbbells), some weight and a bench is all you need to be able to perform dozens of different exercises in your house.

Cons

1. Usually it is harder to learn at first. Especially when compared to machines (and to a lesser extent, body weight exercises), it's usually a little harder to learn proper technique as a beginner.

2. Higher potential risk of injury. There is a risk of injury with EVERY type of exercise, but the potential may be a little bit higher with free weights than others.

2. Body Weight Exercises

A body weight exercise is any exercise where the resistance is provided by your own body weight. Instead of moving a barbell or dumbbell from point A to point B like you would with a free weight exercise, a body weight exercise requires moving your own body from point A to point B. Some common examples include push-ups, pull-ups, chin-ups, and dips.

I see a friend buy exercise equipment and never use it. I think the most exercise they got was when they assembled these machines for the first time. Learn to use your body before you invest in buying an exercise machine.

Pros

1. Completely natural movement. Allows you to move through a range of motion that is completely natural for your specific body. Nothing is restricted or put into any sort of fixed position that may not be perfect for your body.
2. Uses additional muscles. Since you are in full control of the weight (which is your body) and stabilizing the entire movement itself, you are therefore recruiting the use of various stabilizer muscles that tend to go unused with machines.
3. Extremely functional. Body weight exercises allow you to mimic actual movements that you actually do in real life, and in the exact manner you'd actually do them.

Cons

Sometimes too hard/impossible. For certain people (especially beginners and people who are overweight), body weight exercises like pull-ups and dips are extremely hard and, in some cases, just impossible to do. With free weights or machines, if it's too heavy, you can just use less weight. With a body weight exercise, you're kind of stuck with your own body weight. (I will mention however that there are ways around this issue to some degree, but that's a topic for another time.)

3. Machines Exercise

A machine exercise is any exercise that works on a fixed path with the weight (and usually the entire movement itself) stabilized for you by a machine.

Rather than holding the actual weight that is providing the resistance and moving it from point A to point B (like you are with free weight exercises), you are instead holding handles that are in some way attached to some form of weight, and you're moving that from point A to point B.

Some common examples include any type of machine press, row, curl, extension, leg extension curl, and leg press.

Pros

1. Usually easier to learn and do. Using a machine is usually as simple as sitting down, grabbing the handles and moving them in the only direction they are capable of moving. Especially in the case of beginners, this is the easiest form of exercise to learn.

2. Can sometimes be safer. While you can definitely still get injured using a machine, there is usually less risk of injury when compared to free weight or body weight exercises.

Cons

1. Unnatural movement path. A fixed, unnatural movement path forces you into positions that in many cases are not right for many people. At best this can be uncomfortable and might make it hard to progress and properly train the target muscle. At worst, it will eventually cause an injury.

2. Least functional type of exercise. The carryover between machines and movements you actually do in real life is lesser than it is with either free weight or body weight exercises.

3. While you are definitely still working the target muscle and moving the weight (or in this case, the handles) from point A to point B, the entire movement is being stabilized by the machine itself and therefore preventing you from using various stabilizer muscles.

4. Not ideal for home use. Machines are the most expensive (by far), take up the most space (by far), and are the least usable (one machine is typically only capable of one exercise, whereas a barbell or dumbbells can be used for dozens).

Which Type of Exercise Is Best for You and Your Goal?

In most cases, most of the time, this is how it breaks down based on your specific goal:

Performance Related Goals

If your primary goal is performance related (increasing strength, improving performance, etc.), then the majority of your workout routine should be comprised of free weight and body weight exercises. Machines should usually be kept to a minimum, or possibly none whatsoever.

Aesthetic Goals

If your primary goal is looks related (building muscle, losing fat, getting "toned," etc.), then really all three types of exercises can serve as suitable choices for your workout routine. In general, however, free weight and body weight exercises are the ideal first choice, with certain machines being a perfectly fine secondary option.

CROSSFIT: Try the CrossFit's Murph

1-mile run, 100 pull ups 200 push-ups and 300 squats and 1 mile run as a finisher. Let me know about your time at twitter @coachmanjeet if you're not shy and I will give a shout out for you on my social network.

1 MILE RUN
100 PULL-UPS
200 PUSH-UPS
300 SQUATS
1 MILE RUN
"MURPH"

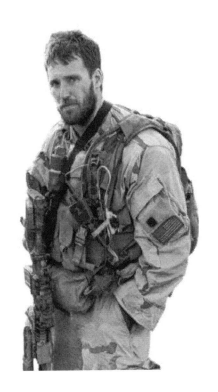

Time Under Tension (TUT)

Although you have read the above article, science claims that irrespective of the weights, your muscles develop when they are put under tension for a certain duration which crosses your muscles threshold. For e.g. You can lift a 20 kg dumbbell and do 5-8 reps, or you can hold a 10 kg dumbbell facing upwards

and hold it for a minute. So, which one is difficult? Which one will give you more benefit? The light weight or the heavy? As both the weights will put your bicep muscle under immense tension for a certain duration. Food for thought! Next time

someone asks you in the gym to lift the heaviest possible weight, ask them to hold the smallest possible weight against gravity for certain duration.

Now that you don't need to bother about lifting heavy or light, let's move on to some personal tips from my own experience. For me it's a mix of heavy and light weights. I will do a heavy weight session at 4-6 rep range followed with a lightweight (not as light as you might be thinking *wink*) session at 8-10 rep range, alternating weekly.

Follow these tips for optimum results:

- Use drop-sets and supersets as tools for more volume in workout. Volume is all that matters.
- Personally, I'd do more incline chest press as it will build your overall chest
- Volume is the key. Instead of doing 4 sets of 12-15 reps, try doing 6-8 sets of 4-6 reps each
- Form is everything. For example, try to retract your shoulder blades when doing chest press. This will minimize the load on your shoulders and maximize the load on your chest.
- Follow a 1:3 approach, 1 second to pick the weight up and 3 seconds to bring it down slowly. Do it slow and do it with proper form
- Use dumbbells wherever possible instead of barbells. It will isolate each side.
- Weighted pull-ups are one of the best exercises; do it every day. Even if you are able to do one, do it with strict form.
- Try to avoid exercises which could hurt your neck, Lat pulldown behind neck is a big no-no. Do heavy lifting, but not ego lifting.
- Use compound movements. Focus on your negatives and try to hold the weight. Build Mind-Muscle Connection.
- Don't overlook calves and hamstrings. You're going to get a lot of negativity if you don't focus on them, especially the calves.

Compound or Isolation: What builds muscle better?

A compound exercise is a multi-joint movement that works several muscles at one time like a squat, which moves both your hip and knee joints and engages your core, glutes, quads, hamstrings and calf muscles. Isolation exercises target one specific muscle group – like a barbell curl working your biceps.

There's a lot of debate about which is best for muscle building, but here's why you need both in your training.

COMPOUND: The foundation of your power

If you're a beginner, compound exercises help you build your foundation quicker by giving you more for the time and effort you put in. They help you lift heavier loads and build more strength overall. Let's talk benefits:

1. They'll save you time. Think about exercises like squats, clean and press, push-ups, and pull-ups. You could incorporate just two of those exercises into a workout, do 10-12 reps in five sets, and have a great full-body workout because you're utilizing the multiple joint movements. To hit all of those muscle groups one by one would take much longer.

2. They're super effective. The more muscles you engage, the more testosterone your body releases. More testosterone means you're capable of more muscle growth. Think of a squat, where you're balancing the barbell on your traps. You're using your torso and core and you're engaging your shoulders, legs, glutes and stabilizer muscles to balance that weight as you bring it down and up. So that compound movement increases your growth factor, allowing your body to really build up power and strength.

3. They'll increase your functional fitness. You're doing compound movements every day: reaching up to get something off the top shelf, squatting down to

pat your dog. Adding functional exercises to your training will help you move easier through life. Plus, getting all-over strong will help you lift more weight in isolation.

ISOLATION: Your muscle building companion

Isolation exercises still have an important part to play in a well-balanced muscle-building regimen. That's why I've added cable machine moves into my newest workouts to help you target specific areas – and make use of that fancy gym equipment. So, why should you do isolation exercises as well?

1. They help target spots you might have missed. Some muscles need isolated exercises. For example, the bicep is used in a lot of pulling movements – for example rows and pull-ups – as a secondary or supporting muscle rather than the primary one. There isn't a compound exercise that can really target the bicep on its own.

2. They'll keep you active all over. If injury strikes or your muscles need time to recover from a tough workout, isolation exercises allow you to work on individual muscles while avoiding those that are overworked or injured.

3.They're perfect for fixing imbalances. We've all got one – whether it's biceps that won't bulge or pecs that won't grow. Isolation training lets you zero in on a muscle and bring it up to speed. In my new workouts, cables help to connect the mind with that muscle, so you can sharpen and fine-tune.

CARDIO

Cardiovascular exercises or cardio are basically any exercises that can raise your heart rate. They are beneficial for your overall cardiovascular health i.e. your heart and your respiratory system. Cycling, running on a treadmill, or crossfit trainer are a few examples of cardio. Cardio can be done once or multiple times throughout the week. However, doing cardio for weight loss is not a suitable option for multiple reasons.

Research has shown doing regular cardio can significantly improve your cardiovascular health; however, it should not be used for dropping inches off your body. From my personal experience, weight training is the best way to do it. Also, fat loss, like we discussed, is a matter of calories in vs calories out. So, revisit your diet.

HIIT Vs Steady State Cardio

HIIT or high intensity interval training is basically a training split in which your resting periods are smaller. An example would be to run on a treadmill for two minutes at 15 kmph and then taking a gap of one minute and then running again. HIIT assists in gaining muscles and is shown to increase your metabolism over a 24-hour period. HIIT is fueled by both glycogen and fat and will not target fat immediately. Some researchers have proved however that doing HIIT will help you reduce more overall calories in a short amount of time than steady state cardio. The scientific logic for this is EPOC. (No in the scope here).

Fitness and workout basics for beginners

Nowadays, more and more people pay attention to healthy life which means to have a healthy mind in a healthy body. We are trying to keep the balance between physical health and psychological well-being. These two are very important. And we have talked a lot about psychological well-being, about how to set our minds and willpower. Now when we know all about it and have practiced it, we should start studying and practicing how to have a healthy body.

Fitness and workout are the only ways to be healthy, strong and beautiful. And as we discussed earlier focusing and concentrating is a must for achieving your every goal, especially fitness and workout goal.

So, make a strong decision and have the grit to do it. Without it, you won't be able to achieve your fitness & workout goals.

Keep a note of how your body feels during exercise and after exercise. Exercising affects nearly every organ of your body. If you exercise a few times a week your body is getting used to it, so you are able to do it more efficiently. And think of all the benefits physical activity has.

Energy to burn

Your muscles must have fuel for exercising. And the fuel comes from the food you eat. The energy is stored in the food in a variety of forms: proteins, fats, and carbohydrates.

Each cell of your body has one primary source of energy which is called adenosine triphosphate (ATP). And your capacity for physical exercises is determined by your body's ability to create ATP. And the reverse is also true: your physical activities determine how well you can generate ATP.

When you are exercising the demand for ATP increases, your body must churn out more. To do this, your body tries to find fat and glucose in different places of your body.

When you engage in physical activity, your body doesn't rely solely on one process or the other; both are used to generate ATP, but one more so than the other. Because of this distinction, exercise is classified into two broad categories, aerobic and anaerobic, depending on which process is predominantly used for ATP production. If the intensity of exercise is such that your lungs and heart are able to supply oxygen for energy production, then the activity is almost exclusively aerobic. But if intensity rises so that the demand for oxygen outstrips supply, then the activity becomes anaerobic.

Walking, jogging, cycling, or swimming at an even pace are aerobic activities. Activities in which your body tends to go anaerobic more quickly include wind sprints and weightlifting.

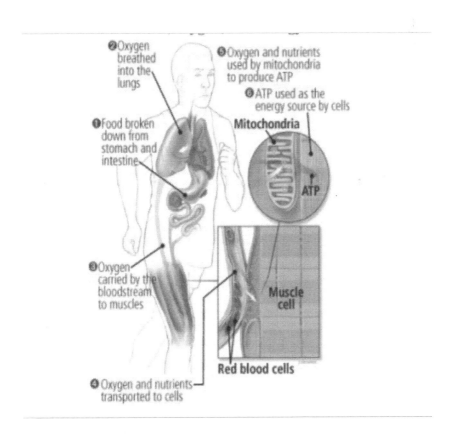

Let me address some common questions first:

1) Do I need to count calories?

When breaking down a bodybuilding diet, macronutrients are often split into percentages. For instance, an off-season dietary recommendation might be to get 50% of calories from carbs, 30% from protein and 20% from fats. To do this accurately, you have to have this valuable information: every gram of carbs has approximately four calories, every gram of protein has four calories and every gram of fat has nine calories. This calorie differential explains why bodybuilders, even those who are not on a low-fat diet, need to pay attention to fat calories, as well as to carbs and protein. For gaining mass, shoot for at least 20 calories per pound of body weight when getting lean, cut calories to 15 or less per pound of bodyweight.

2) How frequently should I exercise?

Allow at least 72 hours between workouts for most body parts (except calves and abs). So, if you train triceps on Monday, you can hit them again on Thursday.

Cardio can rob your recuperative reserves. Avoid leg-intensive cardio the day prior to leg day.

3) How long should I rest?

Well, it depends: If the goal is to slash the fat then your rest should be minimum 90 seconds.

If you want to build mass, rest between 2 to 4 minutes. If you are doing a compound exercise like a squat or deadlift or chest, rest at least 2 minutes.

4) How many reps to do?

Heavy Exercise: 5-8 reps.

Mid compound: 7-10 reps.

Isolation: leg extension- 10-15 or higher. Moderate weight and higher repetition. First, do the compound lift and then move to isolation workout. Abs and Calves are exceptions to these.

5) How much should I lift?

Heavy weight is not important. What is important is whether you are firing the targeted muscle or not. I have seen many folks in the gym lifting very heavy, but they do not gain the size, because they are using the swing to lift the weight. To gain muscle size, you need to break the muscle fiber to trigger the growth. And to break the muscle fiber you need to lift as much as you can control during negative motion (for example while coming down). One way to know the weight is too heavy or not is to count 1, 2, 3 while coming and make sure the weight is in the proper control.

The importance of the right diet

"One of the great moments in life is realizing that two weeks ago your body couldn't do what it just did".

One of the most important things to succeed in fitness for beginners is the right diet. You should know how to cook, how to prepare all your meals in advance, how to count calories, carbs, fats and protein. Many people waste years in the gym and never get any result. They don't realize that no workout works if the food is not on the point. And it's not that hard to manage your diet. You just need to build a good habit.

A good motivation to go to the gym: why gyms try to attract people who won't come?

Most of the gyms can hold only 200 people at a time but how can they still sign up ~5000 + members?

It's simple, they know that only a few % of people will show up. In fact, gyms are trying to attract people who will not come. Normally, we hate being linked with long-term contracts, but gym memberships are an exception. "Joining a gym is an interesting form of what behavioral economists call pre-commitment," says Kevin Volpi, director of the Center for Health Incentives and Behavioral Economics at the Wharton School.

Do you feel bad that you have a yearly membership, but you don't go? You should not because you are helping others who do go.

If everyone who had a gym membership showed up at the gym, it would be a stamped situation. If you are not going to the gym, you are actually the gym's best customer. The reason that gyms can charge so little is that most members don't go. People who don't go are subsidizing the membership of people who do. So, if you don't work out, you are making gyms affordable for everyone.

Workout for beginners

You want to get in shape, but you have no gym membership, or you are traveling, busy, kids, family, more excuses.

That's fine, you don't need a gym and long hours to get in shape! You can work out anywhere in 20 minutes.

Here I am introducing a workout that is good for beginners. But note, this workout will make you sweat like a pig and feel sore all the next day. If this is the first time for you, be careful and don't take big risks.

How to warm up like an Athlete

We have talked about the importance of a good warmup and noted that it is a must before any kind of workout or sports. But what lots of people do is static stretching before the exercise which actually limits their performance and can lead to injury.

From the last few years, I have completely moved away from static stretching to dynamic stretching before starting my all types of different workouts. Whenever I do my full dynamic workout movement, I feel more energized and fully warmed up for my strength training or HIIT training session. If you are going to static stretch, better to do so afterward.

Let's quickly look at the difference between static and dynamic stretching.

1. Static Stretching. Holding a pose without movement for a period of time. Typically, what most people do before a run or workout or what is practiced in yoga.

What is the problem with static stretching if you do it for your workout warmup?

1. Static stretches do not warm up your muscles and cold muscles are more prone to injury.
2. Static stretching does not put your muscles in the right mood to exercise, they relax you.

2. Dynamic Stretching. Offer a warm-up of muscles, ligaments, and joints through movement and is highly recommended prior to any type of exercise.

Here are activities for dynamic stretching

Focus on Rotational Movements

1. Head and Neck rotations in both directions.
2. Trunk rotations and bent trunk rotation (spine straight).
3. Arm and shoulder rotations - small circle and a big circle.
4. Overhead Arm Swing (helps runners, who often have a complaint of back, neck and shoulder issues).
5. Cross extensions warm up – opposite leg and arm movement (this warms up the muscles used when running since you run with opposite arm movement from your legs).
6. Hip rotation – high knees.
7. High leg swing – straight leg (back straight) (don't reach and touch, this puts a strain on the back).
8. High leg – bent leg touching the butt.

Aerobic Movements:

1. Jumping jacks or skipping.
2. Lunges to jumping lunges.
3. Squats to jumping squats.
4. Calf jumps.

Touching the floor and spine movement

1. Indian style push-ups.
2. Cat and Camel. This movement will prolong the life of a healthy spine by hydrating the disks.

Super Slow Resistance Training Benefits

This is a workout where you do the movements at a super slow rate of 10-90 seconds per repetition as opposed to the normal 2-4 seconds per rep. This workout has been proven to give you more results in a shorter time than any other workout when it's done properly.

This is mainly because you are working three muscle fibers at once: slow, intermediate, and fast twitch muscles. Most weight training only works slow twitch muscle fibers, so for most, you are working a group of muscles that is rarely used, allowing you to gain big results fast.

This workout can hit all three muscle fibers, because it's based on high intensity which overrides the normal way of hitting fast twitch which most people do with speed. But it's a misconception that speed is the only way to hit that.

You feel an incredible burn with this as if you are working a muscle you have not worked before in your life and it happens every time you do this but especially in the beginning. This is a breakthrough workout for athletes; people who are looking for a change in their workout, and even people who never work out and want to gain fast results.

So, let's define the benefits of slow resistance training.

15 Minutes to Complete. This whole workout takes under 15 minutes, which sounds ridiculously short but after doing this properly you will not want to do or be able to do more.

Very Safe. This workout is also extremely safe and has very low impact on joints and anyone can do it. In fact, this was originally created for women suffering from osteoporosis to create a safer movement, when the researchers noticed in a short time, they had 50% gain in muscle.

About 30% increase in strength in 6 to 8 weeks. One of the main advocates of this workout named doctor Doug McGuff writer of body by science, says he brings about a 30% increase in strength in 6 to 8 weeks using this routine and almost guarantee a 100% increase in 8 months to a year, and with no injuries, because it is very little force against you, which is what causes joint injuries.

Benefits for organs and heart. This workout also has serious benefits to your organs and heart, YMCA fitness researcher Dr. Wayne Westcott says this pushes more blood to the heart than aerobics and found 50% gains for those working out in this program in 2 months.

Only Necessary to do Once a Week. Another great thing about it is you can do it as little as just once a week. That's because slow twitch muscles, recover very fast, requiring you to work them out 3 – 5 times per week in order to have growth, but fast twitch muscles fibers take 3 – 7 days to recover, allowing muscle growth to occur. In fact, doing it 3 days a week will inhibit growth hormone and raise cortisol levels.

How to Stop an Energy Crash During the Day?

Have you ever heard about the Glycemic Index? Let's understand what exactly it is.

In basic terms, it shows how fast or slows your blood sugar rises after consuming a certain food.

Foods with high GI markers are easily digested and easily absorbed and they create a rapid blood sugar increase. However, foods that are low in GI are slowly digested and take longer to absorb, which means blood sugar will rise a lot slower.

Low GI foods have many benefits in terms of weight management, they help with appetite and diabetes. The low GI diet is considered to reduce insulin levels and insulin resistance.

Now I must point out that a food that is low in GI does not necessarily mean it's a healthy food!

If you consume white bread (High GI Food) with peanut butter, then blood sugar won't rise as much as if you consume the bread alone. This is due to the fat in the peanut butter, the fat content slows it down.

Let's take a look at a scenario.

As we sleep, sugar level drops. If you get up in the morning and don't eat breakfast, blood sugar will continue to drop. And if you don't eat within three hours, your brain tells you, "hey, give me some food". You eat a baguette with some jam on it because it's quick and easy. In this instance, your blood sugar shoots up fast and within the hour comes crashing down, which means by lunchtime your blood sugar will still be pretty low. So, your body will once again ask for some sugar and you will give, which will then give you another big rise in blood sugar. And in the afternoon your body will still ask for some sugar again, so the biscuits come out, yum!! By dinner time your brain will be going crazy asking for more sugar, so you give again and go to sleep.

This keeps happening every day, you are gaining weight, and diabetes is on the horizon!!

Now, do you realize how important it is to know which food gives you a sugar spike and which one does not?

Learn to listen to your body.

Before listening to the health experts on the Internet, learn to listen to your body. Not all health advice works for everyone. Studies with conflicting results are a frequent occurrence. If you don't listen to your body, you might do more harm than good to yourself. When you come across something significant, pause and take time to consider how to apply your learning straight away — within the next 1–3 days.

Your Body's Set Point and Benchmarks:

Here are some baseline benchmarks for being strong and capable. For some they'll be lifetime goals. Others will have long past them.

- Squat: 1.5x BW (bodyweight)
- Deadlift: 2x BW
- Bench: 1x BW
- Press: .75x BW
- Pull-ups: 10
- Push-ups: 55 in 2:00
- 5-mile run: 40 mins
- How do you measure up?

How to recover from an intense workout?

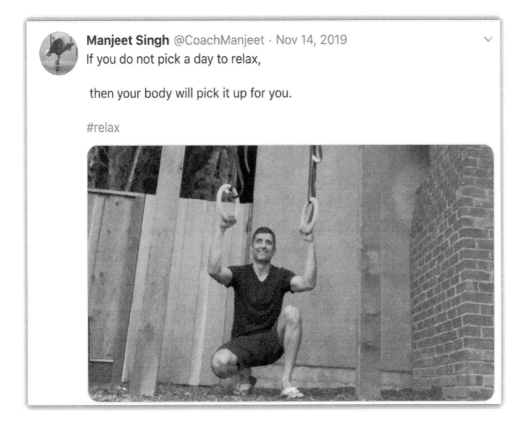

Manjeet Singh @CoachManjeet · Nov 14, 2019

If you do not pick a day to relax,

then your body will pick it up for you.

#relax

I know that you will be very tired from a workout and these tips will be extremely helpful for recovering from an intense workout.

- Eat more carbs and protein.
- Take BCCA.
- Foam Roll.
- Ice Bath.
- Use a tennis ball or Swiss ball.
- Take a small nap during the day.
- Do light workout.
- Take multivitamin.

Good Pain vs Bad Pain: how to reduce soreness?

Maybe you have heard the expression: "No pain, no gain," but that's not always a great rule to follow and the thing is not always about the physical pain. When you are working out alone without a trainer, it's important to listen to your body. If something doesn't feel right, don't push it - your body is usually trying to tell you something.

Good Pain

Though it will be difficult for you to go up and down the stairs, some muscle soreness is normal. This is a good pain, as long as you're feeling that soreness in the places that were targeted during your last work out. In other words, don't be concerned when you wake up the next day after a hard workout feeling a little tight and achy. You're likely experiencing DOMS (delayed onset muscle soreness).

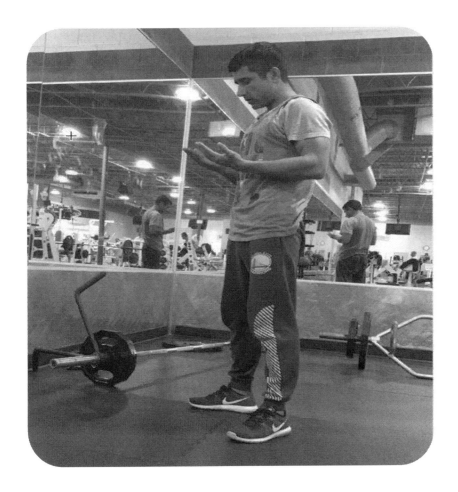

Here is how you can recognize a good pain.

1. Mild discomfort is part of the exercise process and is necessary for the improvement of performance and physique.
2. The burn is a good pain. It should be short-lived and felt only during the exercise.
3. Fatigue after a workout should leave you exhilarated but not exhausted. Fatigue that lasts days means you have been excessively challenged and your muscles and energy stores are not being replenished properly (or diet has not been taken care of). Chronic fatigue is referred to as over-training and is not good.

4. Soreness is common, especially for muscles that have not been exercised for long periods of time - or when you perform an exercise that you are not accustomed to. Soreness typically begins within a few hours but peaks two days after exercise. This is referred to as delayed onset muscle soreness and is normal when beginning a new fitness program.

Bad Pain

Bad pain is usually caused by the improper execution of an exercise. The right exercise shouldn't really hurt. Immediately notify your trainer (if you have one) or a physician of any sharp or sudden pains, swelling, or any unnatural feelings in your joints or ligaments.

Here are some examples of a bad pain

1. Pulled Muscle. If you feel a sudden tightening during an exercise, you've probably pulled a muscle and how you should respond depends on the severity of the pull. Again, this could be a sign from your body that you're overdoing it or that your form is off. Take a break from that particular move or activity until the muscle recovers. You can tell if a muscle pull is more serious if it bothers you even when you move gently, or if the pain persists longer than two weeks. If that's the case, make an appointment with your doctor.

2. Achy Joints. If you're doing a kettlebell swing and all of a sudden you feel a sharp pain in your back, it's time to stop. Soreness or achiness in your joints can also be a warning that your muscles aren't absorbing the force properly and that the soft tissue around your joints (tendons, retinaculum, and musculotendinous junction, for example) is absorbing too much force.

3. Pain that increases. Any kind of pain (sharp, dull, or otherwise) that progressively gets worse, and more intense during your workout is bad news. If you experience any of this, take a break from activity until you can get to your doctor and have it checked out.

Here are 5 Tips to Relieve (or avoid) Sore Muscles

1. Warm Up. Increase body temperature by doing dynamic warmup to help prepare your muscles for the shock of an intense workout.
2. Stay Hydrated. A lack of electrolytes can make muscles sore. Drink a full glass of water after 30 minutes of workout. If you are dehydrated, then drinking water during a workout is not that helpful because it takes a minimum of 20 minutes for the body to use that water.
3. Do Cardio - at the end of a heavy workout. A cardio workout increases blood flow and acts as a filter system. It brings nutrients like oxygen, protein, and iron to the muscles that you've been training and helps them recover faster. As the blood leaves the muscles, it takes some of the metabolic bi products with it (like carbon dioxide and lactic acid) that may be causing DOMS.
4. Foam rolling. Spend at least 5 minutes on a foam roller on heavy workout days. This is a great way to reduce soreness and relax the muscle at the end of a workout.
5. Ice Sore Muscles. Have a cold pack handy to reduce pain and inflammation.

It is recommended to perform each exercise with NO WEIGHT to familiarize yourself with the movement pattern and to mentally and physically prepare you for the tasks ahead. Warming up is a crucial part of injury prevention and prepares your body for exercise by lubricating your joints. It is counter-productive to train through soreness.

"STRENGTH DOESN'T COME FROM WHAT YOU CAN DO. IT COMES FROM OVERCOMING THE THINGS YOU ONCE THOUGHT YOU COULDN'T" – NIKKI ROGERS.

How do I get a six pack? The most common question for those who start fitness and workout.

First of all, you should lose body fat. Losing weight is not the same as losing fat. Weight can come off in the form of muscle, water, waste, and fat. The most effective way to lose body fat is through compound lifts and interval training. After that, abs are made in the kitchen, not in the gym. In other words: eat healthily, work hard.

Basics of Abs

There are basically 2 steps:

1) Get your body fat percentage under 10% (below 17% for women).

2) Build the abdominal muscles underneath.

How long does it take to get six pack abs?

First, you need to know how much body fat you have.

Let's say you now weigh 162lbs.

10.5% x 162 = 17.01lbs of fat.

Now you can calculate your lean body weight.

162 – 17.01 = 144.99.

Let's say 145lbs is lean body weight.

Your goal is to reach 9% body fat. You subtract the goal from 1, i.e. 1 – 0.09 = 0.91.

Now you should divide the current lean body mass by the above figure, i.e. 145/0.91 = 159.34.

So, we can now say that in order to get the six-pack, you need to lose 2.66lbs (162-159.34) of fat. Hardly an arduous task! But we must do it. Here is how.

Do mini cuts: Mini cuts employ a 750 Calorie restriction from the outset. In contrast to a longer cutting cycle, you will perform NO cardio on a mini cut. It is simply not necessary.

How long is it going to take with a 750 Calorie deficit?

As you know, there are 3500 calories in a pound of fat.

2.66 x 3500 = 9310 fat calories.

9310 / 750 = 12.41 days.

That's under 2 weeks to get back in the "very-lean" zone – not bad if you ask me!

Since fat gain should be slow in coming if you eat right 80% of the time, you will probably need to employ a 2-week mini cut every 4 or 5 months. Surely this isn't too much to ask for:

- A year-round six-pack.
- The luxury of allowing some cheat meals every week.

How to be in a caloric deficit without counting calories:

- Don't eat until you're hungry
- Skip breakfast (intermittent fasting)
- Don't snack
- Don't drink your calories
- Eat lots of protein and fats at each meal for satiety

Abs workout

And here is the workout which will help you to get your favorite abs.

- Incline crunches.
- Hanging leg raise.
- Laying reverse crunches.
- Cable crunches.

Shortcuts to 6 packs abs

- Drink two glasses of water before food.
- Get Body wrap - put lotion after shower and wrap overnight.
- Eat more protein, carbs only during the day- protein veggie at night.
- Prepare your own food - make it simple and cook in advance.
- Do both lower and upper abs - contract and engage.
- Use 30 grams of protein after waking up.
- Slow carbs diet.
- Cold bath.
- Bulletproof coffee.
- Beet/Celery juice.
- Do not eat after 7.
- Do HIIT workout and strength training 2 times a week.
- Drink warm water.
- Use spice: cinnamon, red chili, apple cider.

- Define where you have more FAT.
- Ginger and turmeric or pineapple and apple cider juice.

Five golden rules for maintaining abs

Rule 1: Eat like a king in the morning, a prince in the afternoon and a pauper in the evening.

Rule 2: Consume six small meals to keep your blood-sugar levels steady, and 3-4 liters of water a day.

Rule 3: Pack in at least 150g of protein each day from lean red meat, fish, chicken, turkey, eggs, milk, tofu or pulses. Your body uses 20% to 30% more energy to digest protein than it needs for carbohydrates.

Rule 4: Do not stay without food for more than three hours otherwise the body will suppress its calorie-burning capacity.

Rule 5: Don't snack after 7pm.

Food for six pack

- Mushrooms
- White egg omelets or hard-boiled eggs
- Meat, chicken and eggs
- Lean skinless chicken and turkey (white meat).
- Wild Salmon
- Skim milk
- Cottage cheese (fat free)
- Beans, nuts and legumes
- Soy (Tofu)
- Protein drink
- Broccoli

- ⬚ Spinach
- ⬚ Yellow and red peppers
- ⬚ Cauliflower
- ⬚ Sweet potatoes

- ⬚ Brown rice.
- ⬚ Plain Oatmeal (my day starts with it).
- ⬚ Tomatoes.
- ⬚ Berries (extremely high in antioxidants and speed up your recovery).

Six-pack stoppers

Alcohol, white bread, white rice, white pasta, cheese, chocolate, ice-cream, sweets, chips, fries, crisps, soda or soft drinks, fast-food, processed foods/meats (bacon/sausage/salami etc.), butter, margarine, commercial fruit juice, processed & packaged foods.

Increase Your Agility and Flexibility

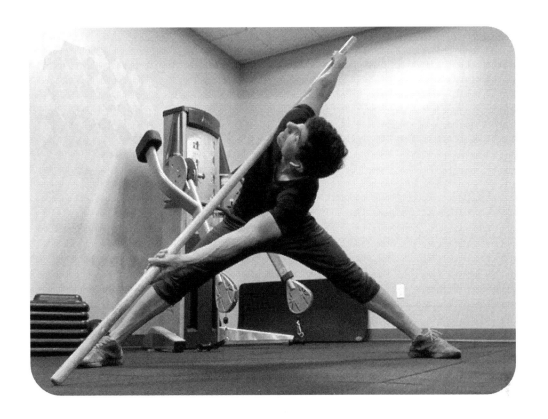

"When everyone is tight, you stay loose. Learn to regulate your body and emotions".

There are many different styles of yoga. All styles of yoga practiced in the west today are variations of Ashtanga, Hatha and Vinyasa.

I have tried many different forms of yoga. There are two particular ones that I really recommend:

1. Vinyasa yoga
2. Bikram Yoga

Vinyasa yoga

Here are few reasons why I prefer this:

- Vinyasa are very fluid, unlike the more static yoga styles such as Iyengar

- Vinyasa actually engages your body like a standard cardio workout
- Dynamic and different. It has a dynamic focus and can incorporate a lot of my fitness workouts within what I do in yoga practice
- Vinyasa yoga is easy to fit into most lifestyles

Bikram Yoga

It was invented by Bikram Choudhury which became popular in the 1970s. Students of Bikram hot yoga perform the same 26-posture series in every 90-minute class in the 105-degree heat.

This is a hot yoga style. Bikram Yoga is usually practiced in a room heated to 35–42 °C (95–108 °F) with humidity of 40%. But to teach an official Bikram class one must be Bikram-certified teachers. They should complete nine weeks of training endorsed by Choudhury. Bikram-certified teachers have a standard way to teach others, but they are encouraged to develop their teaching skills the longer they teach. This results in varying deliveries and distinct teaching styles.

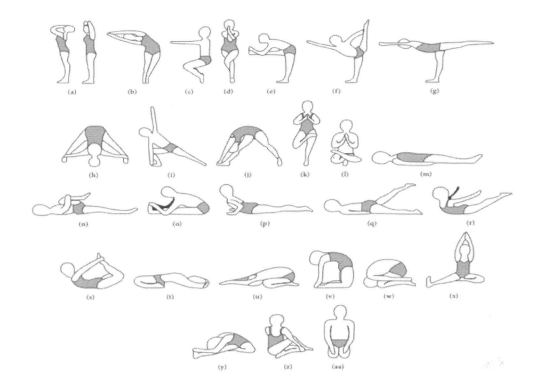

My secret tips for Yoga class

Yoga class is often a reflection of life. Here are my six secret tips that teachers don't talk about very often in class but have really helped my practice.

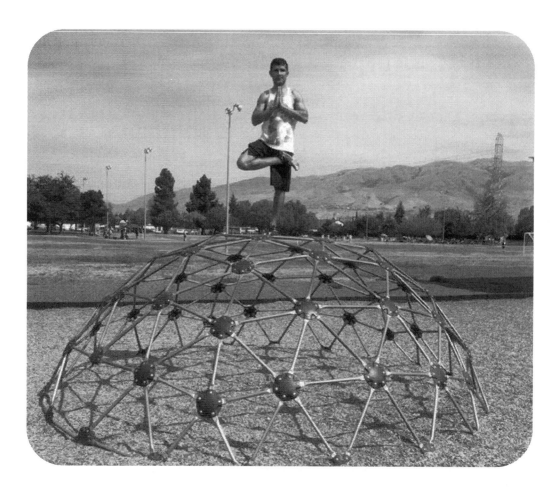

What to Drink/Eat before the Class

Hydrate yourself well before 45-60 minutes of the class. Drinking lots of water just before the class will not help much because it takes a minimum of 20 minutes for the body to absorb water. Avoid eating anything less than two hours before class. Avoid refined foods, such as white bread, pasta and sugar. Excessive consumption of alcohol, caffeine, junk foods and fat also may compromise the quality of your practice. My preference is to have a glass of green juice an hour before the class.

Breathe/Relax your mouth and smile if you feel like it.

Some teachers are obsessed with asking students to smile during class, but I feel strongly that you should only smile if you feel like it. Focus on Relaxing inside of your mouth and Jaw. Focus on deep belly breathing using your nose. Breathe in when you feel the pain and breathe out thinking that the pain is leaving your body.

Endurance and Deep Stretch.

Strive for endurance and intensity in the standing series and focus more on depth in the floor series. The standing series, roughly the first half of class, is intended to generate the internal heat required for you to get deep into your body's organs and muscles in the second half.

Add Strength training to your weekly routine.

Your yoga teacher may tell you that you keep doing Yoga and you do not need any more exercise. For me, I lost too much muscle when I just did Bikram Yoga for two months in a row. I had to get back to strength training two times a week to keep the muscle mass and it also helped in some of the Yoga poses.

Think of stretch and lengthening instead of just coming down with torque.

Use more muscle and less torque. Push yourself but be aware of how much pressure you put on your joints. Know your limits and make progress slowly. Tight Hamstring or Quad: Work on your sit-ups.

To get better.

Practice-Practice-Practice and focus on improving hard poses at home when you have more time and not rushing to finish the pose. Make adjustments - it takes one year to master all 26 poses.

A sample workout plan

> "TRAINING GIVES US AN OUTLET FOR SUPPRESSED ENERGIES CREATED BY STRESS AND THUS TONES THE SPIRIT JUST AS EXERCISE CONDITIONS THE BODY." – ARNOLD SCHWARZENEGGER

A workout schedule that actually works

Here is the new schedule I put together and would stick to it for the next two months. Basically, I have divided it into three parts- A, B, and C. My idea is to cover all three parts at least once a week.

In case of a missed couple of days in between, I would still keep it in this sequence - Workout A, Workout B and Workout C and do not jump from Workout A to C.

Feel free to print it if you find it useful.

Workout A:

Workout A (Legs, Back, Biceps)	5-Aug	12-Aug	19-Aug	26-Aug	2-Sep	9-Sep	16-Sep	23-Sep	30-Sep	7-Oct
Squats										
Lunges										
Lying hamstrings										
Leg Extensions										
CG Pulldowns										
Pullups										
Preacher Curls										
Cable back (squat pos)										
Cable back (one legged)										
Hack Squat										
Hammer curls										

Workout B:

Workout B (Chest, Traps Shlders, Triceps, calves)										
Seated Shoulder Press										
Seated Chest Press										
Dips										
Lying tricep extensions										
Pec Dec (rear delts)										
Seated side delts										
Cable chest fly										
Seated calves										
Shrugs										
Reverse bicep curls										
DB Wrist curls										

Workout C:

Workout C (Core)									
Regular Planks									
Side Planks									
Vacuums									
Captains chair leg lift									
Bicycles									
Leg raises (3-motions)									
Mason Twists									
Sideway Hyperextension									
Woodchops (regular)									
Woodchops (Lo to Hi)									
Woodchops (Hi to Lo))									
Med ball crunches									
Ab-bench									
Oblique side-bend									
	Failed								
	Reset								

Exercise for Muscle Building

First of all, let's talk about the food. You need three types of Macro Nutrition:

- Protein.
- Carbs (Slow carbs, Fast Carbs).
- Fat (Saturated Fat & Avoid Trans Fats).

Your body can take energy from any of these three. Some Carbs are slow digesting. For example- all whole grain items, sweet potatoes. Fast digesting Carbs are white potatoes, white bread etc. Slow digesting foods are not stored as fat.

During a mass-building phase, strive to take a minimum of 2 gram and up to 3 gram of carbohydrates per pound of body weight per day. During cutting phases, reduce total carbohydrate consumption to 1 gram per pound of body weight.

How to increase balance and flexibility?

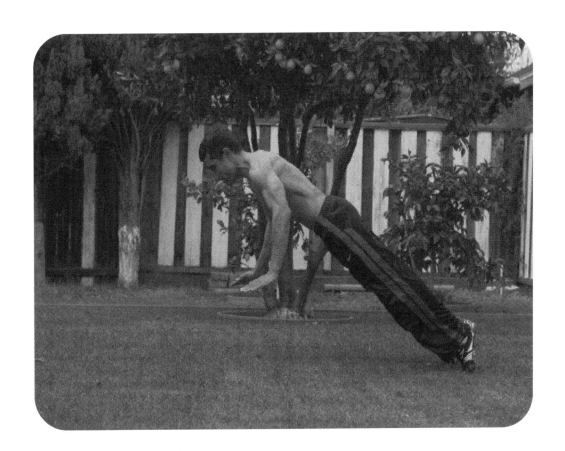

Why is Balance so important?

"Balance is not something you find, it's something you create" - Jana Kingsford.

Balance is the ability to maintain the body's center of mass over its base so that you do not fall. Balance is important and unfortunately, lots of gym-based training avoids it. Most people don't spend any time thinking about their balance until it's too late or when they actually fall or injure themselves. Ask yourself, when was the last time you tried standing on one leg while doing an exercise at the gym, like an overhead press.

Maintaining balance requires coordination of three different sensory systems:

1. Visual system: The visual ability of your eyes to figure out where your head and body are in space, and also your spatial location relative to other objects.

2. Vestibular system: The sense organs in your head, primarily your ears, which regulate your equilibrium and give you directional information as it relates to your head position.

3. Somatosensory system: The nerves in your joints, along with the pressure and vibratory sense information in both your skin and your joints.

Here are my tested tips/strategies to help strengthen the core, eyes, ears, joints to increase your overall balance.

1. Look for things to stand on everywhere around you: sidewalk posts, rails on fences, the back of a bench in the park.

2. Balance on one leg while keeping gaze on something stationary, eventually train yourself to look at objects farther away, then progress to closing your eyes completely.

3. Slowly transition to minimalist shoes (flat shoes).

4. Avoid loud music, loud sounds, and cell phone radiation. These affect your inner ear system.

5. Do side or front leg kicks.

6. Stand on one leg at elevation.

7. When on the computer take breaks and use blue light blocking glasses.

8. Play a sport that requires eye tracking sports such as soccer, golf, tennis, basketball or even ping-pong. These plays aren't only good for training the arm, leg and core muscles you're not using, but also for keeping your eyes on top of their game.

9. Stretching using the ball, balance boards, inflatable balance discs, foam roller.

10. While you're doing day-to-day activities, practice balancing. Try to stand on one foot while brushing your teeth, waiting for a bus or train, doing your makeup or brushing your hair, and other daily activities.

11. Do squats. The first step to improving your overall balance is to strengthen the muscles in your legs, calves, and thighs. This can be done by doing squats on a weekly basis.
12. Close your eyes. You can start by just standing up tall and closing your eyes without moving. Over time, combine the narrow base of support with someone-leg balances while closing your eyes
13. Take a Bikram yoga class or Tai Chi Class.
14. Strengthen your core: Do plank, high knee jumps.

To Sum up: One in three adults over age 65 takes a serious injury from fall each year. The problem is that people are often unaware that their coordination is slipping. Your eyes, ears, and joints are the main elements responsible for providing you balance. Take good care of these elements and train at least 1-2 times in a week to maximize your overall health and fitness training results.

How many days per week do I need to work out?

Depending on your health and fitness goals, you'll need to commit to a minimum of three days of exercise each week to see results. Any fewer than that and each workout will feel like you're starting all over again each and every time.

What are the best exercises for getting rid of belly fat or inner thigh bulge?

Excess fat on the belly, upper arms and inner thighs doesn't typically occur in isolation. If you've got it there, chances are you've got it everywhere. You can't spot reduce. No exercise will target fat cells in just one part of the body. You need to target them all via exercise and proper nutrition.

And if you really want to see muscle definition once the layer of subcutaneous fat is shed, make sure you're following a strength training program designed for muscular hypertrophy (here's where having a personal trainer comes in handy).

How quickly will I see the results of my training?

Expect to FEEL the results of your training sooner than you SEE them. People who start a new exercise program and are consistent in getting their workouts done typically report improvements in sleep, mood and energy levels within two to three weeks. Changes in body composition often take longer to notice; the more consistent you are with your workouts and the closer you adhere to your nutrition plan, the sooner the results will become noticeable (to you and to others too!).

Try focusing on non-scale victories like how many more pushups you can now perform and how your favorite jeans fit.

Why can't I just do cardio?

While cardiovascular training is great for building strong hearts and lungs, it doesn't provide the motivation your body needs to build bigger, stronger muscles and bones. Why? Our bodies adapt fairly quickly to the load we ask them to move; unless you're gaining weight, your legs will always be subject to the same load and moving that load through the same, limited range of motion.

Adding strength training to your program allows you to

- Increase the load on your legs.

- Change the range of motion you move your joints through.
- Target muscles that you don't typically use during cardiovascular training.

Why don't my workouts ever get easier?

You'd think that as your body becomes stronger and more familiar with the exercises, your workouts would start to feel easier. Indeed, many people who 'go it alone' in the gym report exactly this. When exercises are progressed frequently and consistently, the body never truly adapts to the workout, making each feel just as challenging as the one before.

A qualified personal trainer knows how to progress your training plan to keep your body guessing and moving forward at a reasonable pace. When my clients lament that their workouts seem to be just as challenging as they were in the beginning, I know that I'm doing my job well!

Which should I do first: cardio or weights?

While there's some evidence suggesting that if you're doing both in a single session "weights before cardio" leads to faster fat loss, for most people the outcome will be the same regardless of which they do first. If you have a strong preference for one over the other (perhaps you find weights too taxing after cardio? or getting on a cardio machine too boring after you've done your strength workout), go with it. Whatever it takes to get your workout done.

Even better? Make your strength workout metabolic. Add short bursts of cardio-like movement between sets or supersets. Keeping your heart rate elevated while lifting weights is not only more efficient, it may result in a higher calorie burn for the rest of the day.

How long should I rest between workouts?

Rest required between workouts depends on both your conditioning and the nature of your workouts. If you are well conditioned to exercise you may be able to train each day or even twice per day, although almost certainly not the same form of exercise or targeted muscle groups.

If you are new to exercise, particularly resistance work, you should be doing total body workouts to get your body to adapt to the new stress you are putting on it. In this case, I would suggest rest periods of at least 48-72 hours.

Should I walk or jog or sprint?

My answer to the question is that walking, and sprinting are both excellent ways to burn fat. Leave the jogging for running events, not fat loss.

If I stop training will my muscles turn to fat?

This is a very common and understandable misconception. I think it has arisen through anecdotal evidence of big guys who have stopped training and quickly slipped from being muscular to fat. Boxers are a great example. The weight gain is typically because men have become so used to eating large amounts of food when training that they continue the habit even when idle. Combine this with the reduction of calorie expenditure and you're left with a huge calorie surplus every day.

If you avoid eating too much when you stop training, what actually happens is that your muscles lose bulk (they're no longer needed to perform at high levels) but your body fat stays the same.

What is corrective exercise?

Exercise targeting weak areas. One of the most important things you can do for your body is achieve muscular balance. Most things fall into place after that. Imagine each joint as a washer. Your muscles hold that washer in place by providing equal tension on all sides. If then tension is not equal, the joint is unnaturally pulled. This causes compensation and pain. Once your weak areas are identified, implement a program to correct imbalances and help alleviate joint pain. The most common areas reported are low back, neck, hips, shoulders, knees, foot and ankle.

How to Lose Fat and Tone in One Body Part?

There is no magic bullet that you can use to tone up a specific body part and make fat disappear from there. Life will be so much easier if one exercise can actually do the magic in getting the result you want - but unfortunately that does not work. You can't just take the fat and burn it right where it sits; because your body must first convert the fat into a form of fuel that your body can actually burn for energy. FAT is stored all over your body, in some body parts it's more than in others.

Let's look at how the FAT loss works at a high level: when your body needs energy, it doesn't get it from a single specific body part. Instead it will take fat from everywhere and convert it into free fatty acids which enter your bloodstream and become fuel for muscles. That is why it takes more strategic planning if you want to tone a particular body part.

What is an effective strategy to lose Fat and tone in one body part?

- First off all you should find out which part has more fat and focus on that area.
- Consider minimal rest between workout sets, light weight and more repetition.
- Repeat this routine 4-5 times a week.
- Keep an athletic stand while doing exercises and achieve your goal without getting hurt.

Steps #1: Burn phase

- Do 20-25 minutes high intensity/short/Interval based cardio to burn the calories than do toning so that fat gets used for energy.
- I use Tabata songs for my high intensity interval training (HIT).
- I prefer to do the exercise in the morning because your body is already in fasting mode and it will relatively burn more fat.

Step#2: Tone a specific part

- Perform exercises that specifically stress the muscles of the body part that you are trying to spot reduce. (see list of exercise example for toning arms below).

Steps#: 3 Diet

- Reducing your calorie intake by 500 calories daily for seven days will result in 1 pound of fat tissue loss per week, according to the University of Illinois. You'll need to maintain current levels of physical activity, or even increase physical activity, to start burning through fat reserves.
- Fuel moderately. Eat more veggies and high-quality FAT (e.g. Coconut oil, grass fed butter) from morning to late evening.
- In the evening you can have your normal meal but make sure you finish your dinner before 8 pm. The idea is that your food must be digested before you go to sleep.

Example: Exercise List for toning and losing fat from arm

Triangle Push Ups

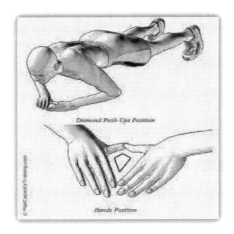

Counter Push Ups

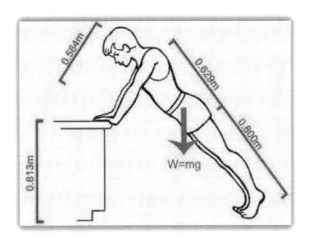

Triceps Kickbacks

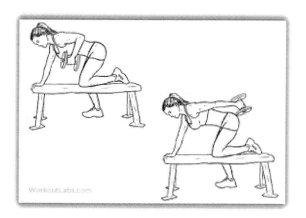

Dips

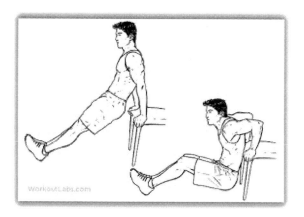

Arm Circle

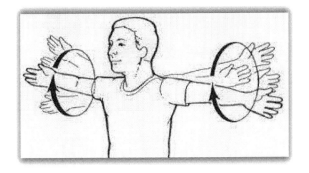

Side planks

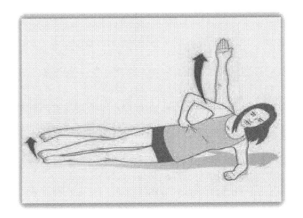

Dumbbell press

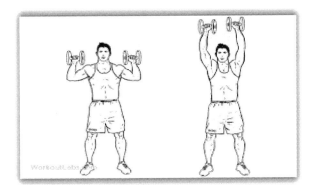

Kettle-bell exercises

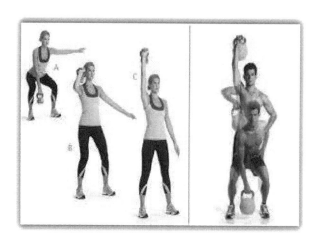

How I found myself doing a 10+ minute plank

Planks are super boring. Who planks for 10 minutes? Well, the official world record is 1 hour and 20 minutes by George Hood. My office's fitness center organizes new Fit-Game challenges every year and this time it was walk the plank. I signed up with two weeks to go.

Plank was never part of my regular exercise regime, and my first day's hold time was 2 minutes. I did some research and laid down a plan to reach at least 8 minutes in two weeks. I made huge strides - increasing my timing by 20 to 30 seconds every day. Today (Feb 25th, 2015) was the challenge day. The last few long planks I have done were around 6 minutes, but I knew that a 10-minute plank was going to happen soon.

I turned on my playlist on the phone, got into position, and the organizer started the stopwatch. There are 20 more people competing at the same time. In the beginning of the plank I had to distract myself as much as possible and keep my mind zoned out. I started enjoying the music --the first song came up in my list "Let's go - Calvin Harris". Who wouldn't get inspired with these words yelling in your ears?

Then I looked at my side buddy on the left. He really started to tremble, and I knew he was going to drop anytime - and boom, he dropped. Looked at the clock and it was somewhere around 5:20. OK- great, I told myself I am halfway done, and I would keep going. Another song came on - "I am the beast", looked in the sides and everyone else had dropped except one guy.

I yelled at myself- how I can drop at this point. I thought of how it would feel to say, "I held a plank for 10 minutes". - And I did not want to have to go through these first 8 minutes again.

The other remaining gentlemen on my right was sweating badly and screaming like he was giving an unmediated childbirth! Who knew just planking could cause such sweat? - that guy dropped around 8.25. I am the only one left and still doing well.

My shaking started, I started to blow out my breath, controlled and strong, and suddenly I was at 9.50. The lady standing in front said- 10 more seconds. And I hold it for another 40 seconds (that brings the total to 10:30).

I am writing about this not because there's anything special about 10 minutes. I'm not stopping here. For people, who are doing a 1 minute or 2-minute plank now – the shaking, muscle burning, sweat, all of this is normal, and it doesn't mean you have to quit. Next time you try a plank, when you think you are done and can't do anymore – hold on for 30 seconds longer. It's not just core strength and stability muscle strength – although these are key – it's that mental toughness that keeps you holding on.

Some Tips I found useful for holding plank longer:

1. Do a little warm up - but do not get tired.

2. Distract yourself by listening to music, watching a video and reading an article, counting backwards.

3. Do not look at the watch frequently - my advice is look only when you start shaking.

4. Breathe- big & deep. Focus on it.

5. When shaking starts- squeeze everything. Flex your quads, tighten your core and squeeze your Tus.

6. Pretend that dropping on the floor is going to crush you and you are stronger than you think!

How to quickly increase Biceps/Triceps Size by 2 inches

I have been working out for years but never really focused on just increasing the arm size. I think the main reason was my satisfaction with biceps/triceps/arm size and I always focused on training the full body.

three months ago, I started to feel that I needed to increase my arm size and made a goal to increase the size by 2 inches. After doing lots of research and trying, I found out that I was not training enough for my arm muscles to grow. Arms are small muscles and they need proper planned and balanced training to grow in Size.

Here are a few things which I learned and tried in the last three months and I was able to increase my arm size by 2+ inches when flexed.

- Dedicate one full workout day to Biceps and Triceps only.
- Train both Biceps and Triceps the same day and then give at least 48 rest before you train them again.
- Focus on BOTH Compound and Concentrated Exercise. Do Superset of biceps and triceps.
- Change Exercise every 2-3 weeks by adding different variations. Sometimes just changing the grip would put the pressure on different points.

- Always do the full motion. Stand in front of the mirror and look from the side to make sure you are doing the full motion. Concentration and correct form are very important to get a quality workout.
- Eat a proper diet including fat in moderation. To increase the size, you need to gain some weight.
- Keep doing some other basic exercises, like squat, bench press and pull-up and chin ups.

Just have an arm day where you blast your biceps with curls, immediately after doing your triceps with skull crushers, do that for around 5 rounds. It would equal like 10 sets. After that do rows or pull-ups followed by dips for another 5 rounds. Every two sets equal a round. I am 100% sure your arms will grow. I always had problems growing arms until I did these workouts. They are military workouts and I guarantee results so long as you keep healthy and do the workouts for about three months. Continue your normal workout regime (shoulder day, chest day, back day etc.) throughout these three months and take your protein after EVERY workout. Finally, be sure to include military press and a demanding full shoulder workout on shoulder day.

Let me tell you that this is not going to be easy - well, if it was that easy then everybody would be walking with an 18" arm. You have to make it a goal, focus on it and visualize very often. You have to be obsessed about getting a big size otherwise you are not going to get it. You will find that you can grow the size by 1" quickly when blood is flowing the muscle but then you will find that it came to the original size if you do not work out for a week. The goal is to increase the size so that 80% of it stays there. It needs patience and time to get the size you want.

Now, I am passing along this challenge to YOU!

Biceps Exercise:

- Barbell curl
- Preacher curl
- Biceps curl - move the pinky out when on top
- Hammer curl
- Seated cable
- Inner grip - works on the outer side of biceps
- Wide grip - works on the inner side

Triceps Exercise

- Skull crusher
- Dips
- Incline triceps
- Close grip chest press

To sum up, here's how to achieve your goals with minimal efforts:

1. Learn how to do high intensity training. Do it for 20 minutes.

2. Do toning exercise for your targeted body part.

3. Buy kettlebell, resistance band, dumbbell and foam roller for stretching (this will be the best $60 spending of your life - trust me!).

3. Eat mindfully. Minimal sugar and processed food. More veggies and high-quality fats.

4. Use your motivation to repeat this for 21 days to convert the routine into habit, and then slowly make staying fit as your ritual.

My exercise routine when my schedule is very busy

I am on an exercise routine from last year, which is a combination of two phases in a week:

Phase One: Hypertrophy and rediscovering the joy of movement.

Hypertrophy is easy. Just focus on the push, pull, and squat. These are the best movements for piling on muscle.

1. Push (The press family): bench, incline, overhead, decline, pushups, and more.
2. Pull (The pull and row family): Any time you seem to be embracing something, that's a pull.
3. Squat: Maximum knee bend with the maximum hip bend. Front, back, Zecher, goblet, and overhead squats.

If the elderly athlete can only do one thing, I would recommend doing the push, pull, and squat three days a week.

WHEN IN DOUBT: KETTLEBELL SWINGS AND FARMER'S WALKS

Hinges are the Olympic lifts, the deadlift, and the kettlebell swing. A hinge is the most powerful thing a human can do.

> *"Practice falling so you won't be helpless when it happens to you"*

Phase Two: Rediscovering the Joy of Movement and Reigniting the Passion

Find an activity that you enjoy, no matter if it's physical or mental.

Do it often to stimulate your body and mind. This is not just about being in a comfortable state, but we also have to learn to suffer for what we love. It could be as simple as sore body parts after training.

I love to explore new body type workouts every week. The learning part of new bodyweight workouts keeps me fresh and entertaining and ignites my passion again and again.

Here is my weekly schedule at a high level, it is easy. I do not feel pressure to do a particular type of workout. I do whatever the mood and energy level is on a given day. I believe in the movement. I do some form of movement every day. Simple!

- 1-2 days of Strength/Hypertrophy training.
- 1-2 days of Mobility/Flexibility drills.
- 1-2 days of Yoga/Breathing/Walking/Playing with my kids.

Why I skip gym often and focused on functional/high intensity interval training

Health and fitness have always been my top priority from school days. I have been going to gym regularly (3-5 days a week) for years, but it has changed about seven months ago. I want to share some information about the reasons I chose to leave my traditional gym type workout behind.

I worked out at the gym for years and was lifting weights a few times a week. It was working well, and I got plenty of muscles and gained strength. But I noticed that I started to get tight over time, I wasn't flexible, and started to get a feeling that it would be hard to continue like this to meet my long-term health goals. There are multiple ways to get the results in the fitness world, but I believe it comes down to picking up something that you enjoy every-time and can continue for years to come. So, I started to experiment with many other options out there, like- MMA, CrossFit, Kickboxing, Calisthenics type, different styles of Yoga, breathing techniques and meditations.

After six months of trial and errors, I currently use a combination of training styles to make sure I am training all my four muscles (Physical, Mental, Emotional and Spiritual) on daily bases. I realized that each of these muscles are important and if one of them is weak, then your life starts to go out of control and balance.

My workout schedules

Here is my typical weekly workout schedule for now.

1. Functional (Calisthenics/Body weight exercises) based high speed interval training (30 seconds full speed and 10 seconds rest, repeat) as the main focus - 3 times a week.
2. Lots of dedicated stretching workout for mobility -> 1-2 times a week.
3. Bikram hot Yoga-> once a week to sweat out extra toxins from the body.
4. Different breathing drills to cleanse the body and control my monkey mind - every morning for about 10 minutes.
5. Meditations -> "Headspace" and "Breath" apps on my phone which guide me to do this for 10-15 minutes every morning.
6. I still have my gym membership and only go there once every two weeks for specific weight training sessions.

I have found that doing body weight training creates a truly firm foundation, helps you be strong while lowering the risk of an injury compared to banging the weight in gym. I am focusing on Calisthenics style combination training because it builds up functional strength, natural looking bodies. And what is more important, you can add lots of creativity to make it fun. With my recent experiments, I found that training for mobility and power rather than muscle size gets you the best result - and some muscle size as a bonus. I am feeling more comfortable and I changed the focus from how I look to how I feel after every session.

Many people seem to be looking for something different, because they are bored of the same old gym/weight routine. It also seems that people want to have more fun when they workout, that is why places like CrossFit has become so popular in just a few years. Functional strength is the strength that you need in everyday tasks, so why not design your training program to focus on that?

Methodologies in fitness are constantly clashing and will continue to do that. Some say lift heavy, others say don't – what to do? You need to experiment with your body/food habits/mind control technique to find out what is working for you. Small changes have started to yield big results for me because I have found my "sweet spot". Find yours. The key is to do the workout you love and do what you can stick with.

Until then, stay focused, safe and try to train all four-muscle every day!

Workout for plus size overweight people

1. Kettlebell swings
2. Leg ups and down
3. Assisted sit on the chair
4. Leg up and down on the table
5. Plank: Start on the wall - on the chair, on knees, and on the floor
6. Trips dip on the chair
7. Side touch
8. Leg up down
9. Beer Squat. The bear squat is the safest variation a client can execute. It uses a Swiss ball which is placed behind the hips, on top of the heels, and against a wall

10. Squat on the chair

11. The landmine squat by Travis Pollen which is much like the goblet squat.

12. Goblet squat

13. Stand holding a light kettlebell by the horns close to your chest. This will be your starting position

Five Body Weight Exercise that everyone must learn

[Note: Do 3-5 minute warm up by doing your favorite moves to open up the joints before you start]

1. Body Weight Air Squat [max rep, 2 sets]

2. Push-up [max rep, 2 sets]

3. Pull-up [max rep, 2 sets]

4. Plank [max hold time, 2 sets]

5. Finish with deep stretching of seven major body parts for roughly 5 minutes

Exercise and the menstrual cycle for women

Can you work out during your period? The answer is "Yes". Generally speaking, working out during your period is a good thing, because exercise helps relieve period-related annoyingness like anxiety, fatigue, and headaches. There are many Olympic athletes who performed at peak during their periods. However, it is important to keep in mind exercising around and during your period is very individual depending on your symptoms, stress micronutrient deficiencies, thyroid problems and the mystery of how variable the menstruation cycle could be.

Here is the good news. You can use these hormonal cycle changes to your advantage by planning and tracking the full mensuration cycle, week by week (considering 28 days cycle here):

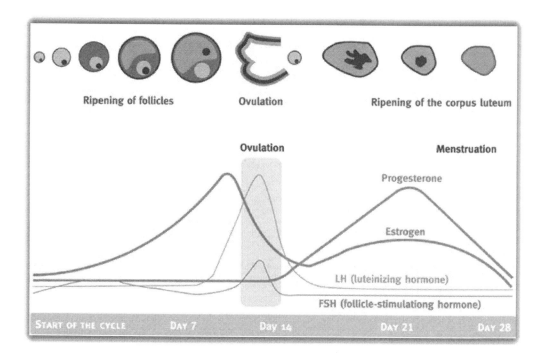

Note: This below recommendation is generic and you should consult a specialist and listen to your body instead of blindly following this advice (or any advice for that matter).

1. Follicular Phase and Menstruating (Days 1-13)

For roughly two weeks before your period, you're in the high-hormone phase. At this point in your cycle, which starts when you ovulate and ends with the first day of your period, your estrogen and progesterone levels peak. You can use this period to your advantage by doing strength training:

Week#1: During this time, recovery time can be quicker and the pain tolerance higher. Make sure you warm up properly because you are more injury prone during this week. Workout option: Yoga, Swimming, walking and light strength training.

Week#2: In Week 2 Your body is preparing for ovulation and hormones are on the rise. The additional estrogen allows your muscles to absorb sugars more efficiently, giving you a little extra energy. This means that you can do a high-intensity workout (like kettlebell swing, burpees) and strength training (lift weights or use resistance bands).

2. Ovulation period (Day 14)

Estrogen is at the highest point, keeping you focused on your body. The best is to do some light warm-up and stretching. Listen to your body - if you have cramps or excessive flow take that day off. If there is not much pain or cramps, then you can do any of the following workouts:

- Walking/jogging/stationary bike (yoga- except inversion poses).
- Use the foam roller and do some light stretching.
- Going up/down the stairs a few times or doing some household cardio work (e.g. prepare food in the kitchen).

3. Luteal Phase (Days 15-28)

When you have your period (and the week after), your body is more like a man's. During this part of your cycle, your levels of the female hormones estrogen and progesterone are at their lowest point.

Week#3: Focus on the moderate workout. Like group classes because you may feel inflamed and bloated. The workout you can do is Pilate, running, power yoga.

Week#4: You can come back to your strength and weight training. This week you can really make progress on your strong side.

What exercises should you avoid during your periods?

Inversions type workout moves aren't recommended during your period, like headstand or any other yoga/exercise pose where your head is down for more than 10 seconds. Why? Because, standing on your head engorges your blood vessels in your uterus, which can make you bleed more. So:

- ▢ Make sure to start with a warm-up to loosen your muscles and joints.
- ▢ Start slowly and progress as your body allows.

What food should you avoid during your periods?

- ▢ Soya: Eliminating commercial soy sources such as tofu and soymilk can help some women avoid estrogen dominance, which can lead to menstrual cycle irregularities.
- ▢ Caffeine.: Avoid the extra stimulant. Drink more water to stay hydrated.
- ▢ Eat healthy, preferably homemade food.
- ▢ Take supplements and pain medication as recommended by your doctor.

Long Distance Running

Got these tips from my friend who is a marathon runner:

Running is all about stepping one foot in front of the other. Sounds easy enough, right? But if your running form is incorrect, you'll end up with aches, strains, and injuries that could prevent you from lacing

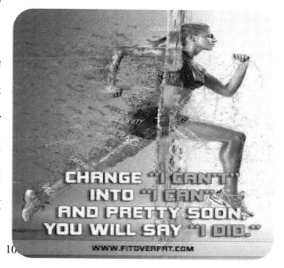

CHANGE "I CAN'T" INTO "I CAN" AND PRETTY SOON, YOU WILL SAY "I DID."

WWW.FITOVERFAT.COM

up your sneaks at all. Make sure to avoid these running-form mistakes the next time you hit the treadmill, trail, or pavement.

1. Head

It sometimes feels good to close your eyes and relax your chin toward your chest, but don't keep your head down (or tilt your head up) for long periods of time. Prevent neck strain and encourage an open throat for easy breathing by keeping your head stacked over your spine. Correct head position also encourages a straight, upright stance, which makes you a more efficient runner.

2. Shoulders

Without even realizing it, you may be running with your upper back and shoulders tensed up toward your ears. (And you wonder why you have a pounding headache or aching neck.) Every so often, take a nice deep breath in and as you exhale, relax your upper torso and actively roll your shoulders back and down toward your pelvis. Do a self-check to make sure your shoulders are stacked over the hips. Hunching the upper body forward not only makes it difficult to breathe, it also puts pressure on your lower back.

I'm just getting started so keep reading to find out what the rest of your body shouldn't be doing while running.

3. Arms

Leave the side-to-side swaying arms for the dance floor. Your arms shouldn't move across your body when you run: it uses up energy, tires your muscles, and actually prevents your body from propelling forward. To increase your speed and endurance, focus on swaying your arms forward and back, keeping your elbows at 90-degree angles.

4. Hands

Clenched fists translate to tense arms and shoulders, which tires your muscles and can cause a dull, achy sensation. Not to mention, it also makes you look like an angry runner! Maintain a sense of relaxation in your torso by running with a slightly open fist, pretending you're holding an egg in each palm.

5. Belly

Many runners complain of lower back pain, and one reason is because they don't engage their abs. While running, concentrate on drawing your navel in toward your spine to keep your pelvis and lower spine stable.

6. Feet

Where your feet strike is a big debate among runners. In order to land with the least amount of jarring pressure on your ankles and knees and have the ability to push off the ground with great force, it's best to land on the mid foot, not on the heel. Then roll forward quickly onto the toes, popping off the ground with each step. Landing softly is key, no one should hear you pounding your feet as you run. Think of yourself as a deer, quietly and effortlessly bounding as you move.

SPIRITUAL FITNESS

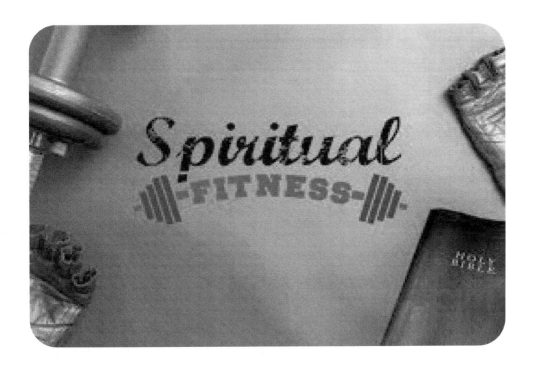

Living with an Ethos and clear purpose

Being successful is all about 'the big picture'. You should clearly define and visualize what is "your mission" and ethos ("values").

One of the fundamental components to having a fulfilling life is having a purpose.

When you have a clear purpose, you know what you are going to do when you wake up in the morning. You know your activities and the path that will lead you to your goals. If you want to go deep and understand what a clear purpose can do for you should read Victor Frankl's famous book, "Man's Search for Meaning".

Having a purpose also gives us a strong feeling of self-esteem. As we feel that we are conquering the challenges and getting closer to our goals we feel more confident and comfortable for what we are doing.

The scientists at Chicago's Rush University Medical Center did many observations and found out that having a goal in life affects cellular activity in the brain. Having a goal increases the brain's protective reserve.

When you know your purpose, you can also clearly define what is important and what is not important for you. And then you will be able to focus only on the important things. Apply the 80/20 rule here and works on the things that help fulfill your purpose.

How to Find Purpose?

- Figure out what you are good at and figure out what you are interested in – those are things you're capable of having passion for.
- If you can get paid for it, then it can serve as a purpose, if not, then it can serve as a great hobby.
- The internet makes a lot of what would have otherwise been hobbies monetizable, thereby increasing the scope for a potential purpose.
- If you choose to live a zombie life – where you drown yourself in continuous entertainment and hedonism, you're going to find yourself depressed and unfulfilled.
- Fulfillment requires self-control and discipline.
- Purpose is not a singular objective. It is a direction and way of life.
- Your life gets meaning as you live in the direction of your purpose.
- The modern world is easy to live in. Comfort will get you nowhere.

Gratitude

No matter what happens in your life, always smile and be thankful for whatever you have. You don't need to have a perfect life to be grateful.

Research has shown that when we are grateful, we are less materialistic and envious of other people. This leads us to happiness and well-being. We also become more forgiving and care about other people.

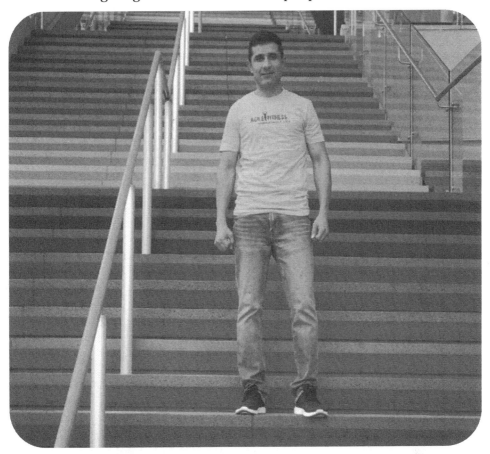

Here is a way to start practicing being grateful:

- Every day I find something to be grateful for.
- Keep a journal and list all the things you are grateful for. Be truly thankful that you have them.
- Practice mindfulness. Look around and notice everything that is worth being noted as beautiful. Be thankful that they exist in your life.
- If you are spiritual you can express your gratefulness in your players. It is the most powerful way to express your thankfulness and deeply feel it.

Powerful morning routines for success

Morning is the most important part of our days because we start a day in the morning and what we do affects our whole day. Waking up and rushing to work is not the best thing to do in the morning. It is better to boost your energy and clear the mind.

So, if we want to be productive, joyful and energetic during the day we should start it appropriately.

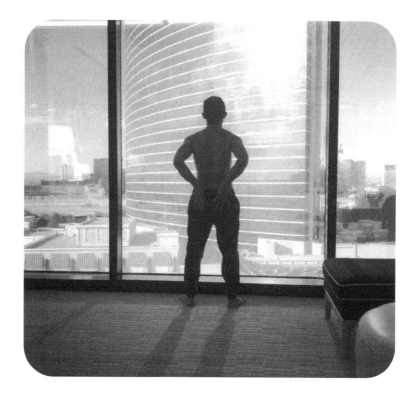

If we want our morning and the whole day to be effective, we, first, should get a good sleep. So, always consider going to bed early. We will talk about the importance of good sleep later.

And the second most important thing is waking up early. This is important because research shows that in the morning our brains are more productive and ready to work.

Actually, knowing and implementing good morning habits is a science and a great art. If you can build your morning routine you will feel more calm, controlled and powerful.

And guess what, the most common and powerful elements of morning routines are very simple and easy. It is just important to turn the morning into a positive experience.

I have done some research to identify what successful people do in the morning. I gathered some of the most important and powerful ones. Here they are.

- Drink a glass of water. Your body and brain need water in the morning.
- Meditate from 6 to 7 minutes. It's a great way to clear your mind and start the day with a calm, clear head. You can either use a meditation app or just sit in a quiet and lit room to practice breathing in and out.
- Bring your attention to love, success and gratitude.
- Make "To Do List". Figure out the priorities and make sure to do those things first.
- Do things to get energy. Working out or moving are very important factors for building energy.
- Have a good breakfast.
- Fill your journal of gratitude.
- Ask yourself one simple question. "What I will do if this was my last day."

Finding hidden Joy and meaning in whatever you do

Everyone wants to find a great love and meaning in whatever he/she does. But usually we do things that we don't love much but those things are necessary to accomplish some important thing.

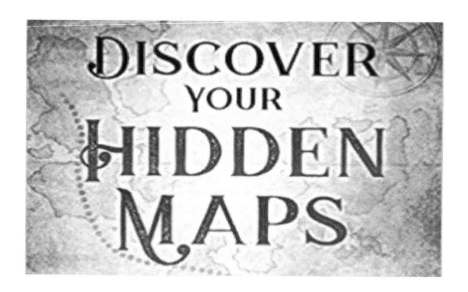

DISCOVER YOUR HIDDEN MAPS

Maybe, it is something that fills your resume or pays your bills. We can do this kind of thing but if they go longer it can be depressing and annoying for us.

The best way to conquer this situation is trying to find hidden meaning and joy in everything we do. Think about all the good things that bring your activity and think about what you will gain from it. Indeed, sometimes you must try harder to find that meaning. Attach that activity to your dreams. It will give you a new drive and energy to do the work. You can also write it down. Write what you are doing now and for what you are doing it. Focus on the results and recognize all the benefits.

Valuing all the little benefits in your life will also help you to find meaning in every moment of your life. Maybe you don't have a much meaningful moment (or you just think so), create it on your own. Don't take anything as it seems to be.

I want to share with you a secret to more happiness, it is helping others. When you are helping you feel more valuable and your time seems to be spent with purpose.

Be happy every moment

"A calm mind equals a happy life."

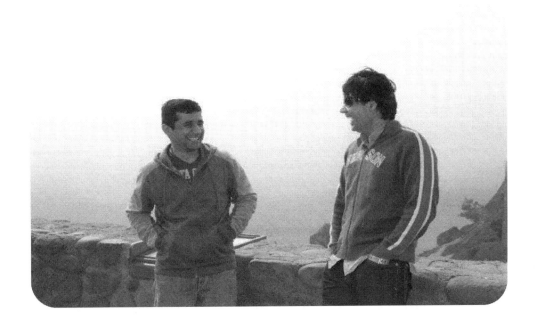

Do you remember, when was the last time you felt complete happiness? Completely free, just enjoying every second.

Yesterday is long gone. Tomorrow will never come. I'm happy today, with my bread, with my smile, with both feet flying in the air. Free like a bird.

My main goal in life is I want to be happy. I want every day to be as smooth as possible. No hassles.

If you want to achieve your goals and live a meaningful life you just must be happy. Happiness gives us strength and joy in conquering our daily challenges and difficulties. When you are sad, just remember all the good things in your life and be grateful for them. Act as a child, find little joy and happiness in everything you see and do.

Don't wait for something to happen or something to change. Feel the beauty and hope at this moment. Be fully present in whatever you do. Then you will be content and peaceful and will live your life in present. Your life is now, and it will always be now. Now is the right time to do what you have always wanted to do.

Here is one unpopular truth.

> *No one in this world is happy for you as much as they say, they are. And no one is as critical of You as they appear, they are.*

Best approach is don't get carried away by extreme emotions!

Comfort will Dull you. Discomfort will Toughen you. Staying at the edge of discomfort is a good strategy.

To me, becoming "AgileFit" means combining practices from both ancient wisdom and modern science. Make continual Improvement your lifestyle.

SECTION 3

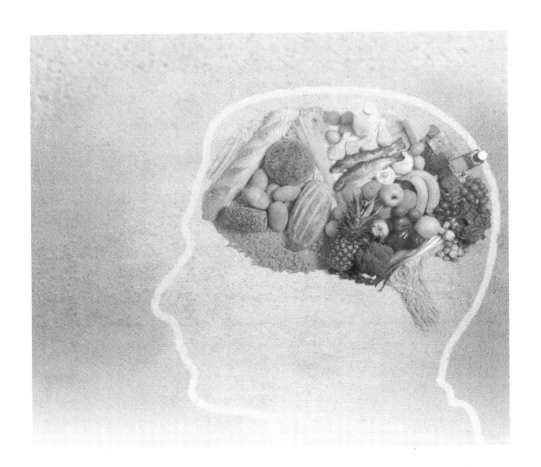

NUTRITION AND

WEIGHT LOSS

Manjeet Singh @CoachManjeet · Dec 28, 2019
We kind of have two brains 🧠 in our body.

1. The brain in your head
2. The "brain" is your stomach.

Make sure you are feeding right things to both. Everyday.

#wellnesstips

Before getting to the details, please understand a few things very clearly:

1. Fitness is science. If you're getting desired results without needing a proper plan for nutrition and workout, then good for you.

2. To lose weight, you have to take fewer calories than your Total Daily Energy Expenditure, to gain weight you have to take more calories than that. Simple and logical.

That's it, and there is absolutely NO WAY around these two guidelines. Let science guide your transformation journey, not bro-science.

NUTRITION

Hard work in the gym isn't something uncommon. Everyone works really hard, and yet they don't get results.

To start with, you have to know your basal metabolic rate (BMR) or your resting metabolism.

Calculating the BMR

First things first, you need to calculate your BMR, I hope you know why we're doing this? If not, please go back and read it again.

ENGLISH BMR FORMULA:
Women BMR = 655 + (4.35 x Weight) + (4.7 x Height) - (4.7 x Age) Men BMR = 66+(6.23 x Weight) + (12.7 x Height) - (6.8 x Age) Weight in Pounds, Height in Inches, Age in Years

Once you know your BMR, you can calculate your Daily Calorie Needs based on your activity level using the Harris-Benedict Equation.

To determine your total daily calorie needs, multiply your BMR by the appropriate activity factor, as follows:

Calorie-Calculation

For sedentary (little or no exercise)

= BMR x 1.2

For lightly active (light exercise/sports 1-3 days/ week)

= BMR x 1.375

For moderately active (moderate exercise/sports 3-5days/week)

= BMR x 1.55

For very active (hard exercise/sports 6-7 days a week)

= BMR x 1.725

Total Calorie Needs Example

If you are sedentary, multiply your BMR (1745) by 1.2 = 2094. This is the total number of calories you need in order to maintain your current weight.

Once you know the number of calories needed to maintain your weight, you can easily calculate the number of calories you need to eat in order to gain or lose weight.

Since our goal is to get shredded, we'll have to reduce our calorie intake. Those looking to gain weight can follow the same routine, except that they have to increase their calorie intake above the Total Daily Energy Expenditure (TDEE).

Remember, if you don't count your calories, your results won't be quantitative and you'll have to rely on hit and trial, so I suggest you do count your calories. Most of the food we consume has labels indicating both macro (Protein, Carbohydrates, Fiber and Fat) and micronutrients content (Vitamins, Minerals).

Lean Mass calculation

Now we all know how to calculate our BMR, but it is to be noted that before calculating the BMR we should know the value of our body fat. Basically, our body fat percentage decides if we need to calculate our BMR by considering our total body weight or our lean body mass. Lean Body Mass is basically the fat free mass in our body. It's also not your muscle mass so kindly don't get confused between the two. Normally if your body's fat percentage is more than 20 (in case of men)/28 (in case of women), it is advised to consider the lean mass to calculate the BMR.

There is a very simple formula that is been used to calculate the lean mass i.e.:

Lean Mass = Total Body Weight – (Body Fat % x Total Body Weight).

For example, if a person is weighing 100 kgs and has body fat % of 40 then his lean mass would be 100 – (0.40 x 100) = 60kgs. So, the above person should calculate the BMR by putting his lean mass i.e. 60kgs instead of total body weight i.e. 100kgs.

Now I'd be giving out my personal diet that worked for me, might not necessarily be working for you.

You know the saying "give a man a fish, you feed him once, teach a man how to fish and you feed him for a lifetime". I am going to do the latter. Many people are going to hate me for this.

I will discuss the following diets. Ratios for the macronutrients (carbs, protein,

fat) are mentioned in the same order. Remember, these ratios aren't the biggest factor in determining your gain or loss of fat. What matters is your overall intake and overall expenditure and the difference is what stays or goes out of your body. However, these ratios and different diets help you follow a diet well, and has other aspects to it:

LOW CARB DIET (25:35:40)

This would be required to trim excess body fat, while making slow lean gains. It is effective, however takes a lot of time to show results (ideal for anyone who's new)

ZONE DIET (40:30:30)

This is the diet that has higher amounts of carbohydrates. This is ideal for the ones who absolutely love carbohydrates. This is also perfect for the people who have high tolerance towards carbohydrates which is commonly seen among the people with high muscle mass.

DEPLETION DIET (DYNAMIC)

To reduce body fat% dramatically and bring definition to your muscles in a very short period (not for people with body fat above10%). This diet focuses mainly towards glycogen depletion and also reduces the subcutaneous water retention to a certain degree.

KETOGENIC DIET (5:35:60)

A ketogenic diet will also target your body fat levels and like the depletion diet, it will also reduce your water retention to a large extent. It engages your body in producing more ketones (will discuss in the diet sections) hence the name, Keto diet. It is an ideal diet to start with if your goal is fat loss but would be sub-optimal for muscle gain.

I will also cover and carb loading. In brief however, since it is a very complex subject and a lot of research is still going on about it.

Before you start planning your diet, you have to calculate your BMR as mentioned before. Figure out how many calories you're going to consume to reach your target goal and then based on the diet, you have to divide your macronutrients into ratios.

REMEMBER, the BMR we calculated above only provides a baseline, many people have the metabolic rate above it or under it and therefore BMR should not be considered a universal indicator of one's metabolic rate.

My Personal Diet Sample

So, by now you must have understood that everyone owns a different car and I have my very own car. In this section, I'll tell you about how I fuel and maintain my car. Note that your car is different, so do not apply these to yourself.

However, here you go!

I try to keep things simple. The taste doesn't really matter to me as long as I am getting the desired results.

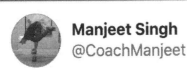

Manjeet Singh
@CoachManjeet

Wellness warriors prioritize health over taste.

9:18 PM · Oct 29, 2019 · Twitter for iPhone

Now some people won't be able to do that. I urge people to start a diet which they can sustain in the long run rather than copying from others for a short period only to eventually give up after getting frustrated.

Here's what I mostly eat:
I use eggs as my staple for protein, brown rice and oats for carbs, and nuts and flaxseeds for fats.

Keep the staple same and you have the flexibility to play around.
For example, if I have to reduce my caloric intake, then instead of eating 100 gm brown rice, I'll eat 50gm, same for protein and fat. Monotony is a part of

the deal, but don't forget, you cannot achieve what you desire for sitting in your comfort zone.

You have to go walk the hard path!

FOOD	CALORIE	PROTEIN, CARBS, FAT
AROUND 7 AM 1 Scoop Protein Shake	121 cals	25gm protein 3 gm carbs 1 gm fat
AROUND 12PM 5 Whole Eggs 1 Bowl Spinach 150gm Mct Oil 1Tbspn Fat Free Curd 100gm	350+80+130+40 = 600 cals	30gm protein, 15gm carbs, 45gm fat
AROUND 3 PM		
AROUND 8PM POST WORKOUT 2 Scoops Protein	242 cals	50gm protein, 6gm carbs 2gm fat
AROUND 9PM 1 Bowl Spinach 150gm Mct Oil 1Tbspn Fat Free Curd 100gm Brown Rice 30gms	80+130+40+150cals = 400 cals	Around 45gm carbs, 20gm fat, 5gms protein
AROUND 8:30PM	220+102 =322 cals	60gm protein, 5gm fat
10 PM Sleep		
TOTAL	1685 cals	170gms protein, 69gms carbs, 73gm fat

You can use the following table to choose your staples.

PROTEIN	CARBS	FATS	FIBER
Chicken	Green Vegetables	Paneer	Vegetables
Eggs	Fruits	Yogurt	Sprouts
Fish	Rice	Cheese	Fruits
Whey Protein	Legumes	Olive Oil	
Tofu	Sprouts	Flaxseed	
White Mushrooms	Banana	Fish Oil	
Paneer/Cheese	Wheat	Nuts	
Soybeans/chunks	Quinoa	Coconut	

This limited list is only for your reference (in no particular order). There are several others you can choose from

How to make a Diet Chart all by yourself

Stop stressing over what diet to follow and how to make a diet chart. There are many resources online, I will give you my favorite ones.

1. Install apps like My Fitness Pal. Google store link / Apple store link.

2. Now while signing up, they will ask you details like height, weight, age and body fat percentage.

3. Go to the BMR tool. Calculate your BMR and TDEE.

4. Now if you want to lose fat, eat less than your TDEE and if you want to gain, eat more than your TDEE. Also, understand, online calculators are just for approximation, keep trying till you find what your maintenance (actual TDEE) calories are.

5. Go to the macros calculator and follow any type of diet, high or low carb. Just be in deficit or surplus as per your goals. Just keep protein intake around 1.8/2g per kg of your body weight and adjust carbs and fats as per your preference. Try to keep fats at least 30-40% of your total calorie intake, rest you can keep carbs.

6. 1 gm protein has 4 calories. 1 gm carbohydrate has 4 calories and 1 gm fat has 9 calories. Now accordingly add food in 'diet tool'. For example, 1 egg has 6gm protein, 5gm fats and 0 carbs, total calories come to 69 calories.

What it takes to eat healthy

If you eat food and an hour later, you are craving again which means your body is not satisfied with what you ate earlier. Focus on consuming nutrition dense whole food and do full meals. Snacking all day messes up your immune system.

If you want to feel good, be healthy and have much energy, the first thing that you should think of is exercising and eating healthy.

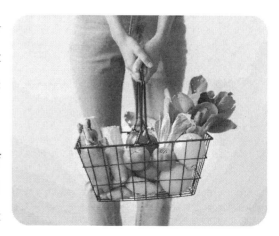

Healthy eating reduces the risk of becoming ill from high blood pressure, high cholesterol, heart disease, cancer, etc.

You may wonder, what is healthy eating. Eating healthy means to get the right amount of nutrients - protein, fat, carbohydrates, vitamins and minerals. They all are necessary to maintain good health.

People get metabolic syndrome by never depleting their glycogen stores; and that is the root cause of many chronic diseases including cancer. Here are some ways help improve or eliminate these issues: Cut sugar, and seed oils, Lift weights, fast intermittently, eat whole food.

Why is eating healthy hard?

Our brain loves sugar (glucose) and when your body has no sugar, you start craving for food.

If you want to get rid of something, you should decide what you will get for it. For example, I am a fan of adding good things (veggie, water, protein...) and focus less on reduction. This applies to food as well as emotional health.

Relationship with Food

I see food as fuel for my body, and it has amazing power to heal any disease or illness. On the other hand, it has the same power to make you sick if you are putting bad stuff in your body.

Some basics first: how do you know what food is good or bad for you? Well, you can say I can Google and make a list. Let me make it simple for you: Keep a record of how you feel after eating all your food for 2 weeks. If a particular food is making you lethargic and bloated (usually all processed sugary food/drinks falls into this category) then do not eat it and then make a list. If something is making you light and energetic then it should be into your "Good to eat" list.

Tips to get started

1. When you go to groceries, buy items that are in your good food list. You may argue that I need to have some crunchy/fried/sugary snacks to treat my guests or for my weekend parties. Here is the solution — pick small limited quantities.

2. Change the environment and keep willpower. Replace bad options with good options. I know you can control yourself even if you have that food around by using your strong willpower. But my point is why waste willpower to control when you can change the environment and save the precious willpower for some other important tasks.

3. Do not leave delicious and unhealthy food in the kitchen or on your desk. Instead keep more plain water around.

4. Setup the environment that works for your lifestyle. You do not need to worry about calories or fat if your ingredients are good and you are limiting sugar and frying in your cooking process.

5. Cook your meals in advance. I know you may be busy and do not have time to cook every day. The solution is to cook 3-5 meals in advance and put them in the refrigerator. Buy Tupperware to store your food and pick a box whenever you are hungry. One more bonus tip: if you are hungry all the time then it indicates that your meal was not balanced. Try adding some more good fat (like grass-fed butter, olive oil, avocados, coconut oil, and nuts).

6. Cook unhealthy food in a healthy way.

7. If you want to eat some unhealthy food, for example, chocolate, eat it in the middle of your healthy meal. Then your mind will accept healthy food at the start and at the end of the meal.

8. Keep away your candy wrapper.

Easy Roadmap to Quit Sugar Consumption

First 24 hours: find times when you are most likely to eat, do something else during that time.

Next 3-5 days: Double your intake of complex carbs

Next 2 weeks: Do not buy: bring sugary stuff at home. Make it hard to find.

Remove Vegetable seed oil from your diet.

We all should replace vegetable/seed oils (canola, sunflower) used at home for a better health with

1. Use Olive oil for low-temp cooking (quick omelet)

2. Use Ghee, coconut oil/Avocado oil for high-temp long cooking.

The key is to know the smoking point temp. of each.

How to eat out without getting Fat

1. Eat a healthy snack at home before you go out.

2. Drink a big glass of water

3. Pick high protein and veggie first

4. if you don't like the taste of something, don't eat it.

5. Do not consume free drinks

6. Eat slowly, learn to chew your food

How to Make Delicious Smoothies that are Healthy

Smoothies are one of the most delicious types of food/drink in the world. But are they healthy? It all depends on how you're making them. Smoothies can be perfect for your dietary goals, but they can also easily get way off, as it's easy to accidentally double something like peanut butter, and all the sudden you have an extra 200 calories!

3.2.1 Rules for Making Healthy Smoothies

1. Don't make it too fruity or sugary. Try stevia or 1 chopped date or every bit of raw honey instead if you need it sweetened.

2. Always have a protein source - so that it will keep you full for hours with energy.

3. Measure your amounts. It's easy to have too much of an ingredient or too little, depending on your goal.

1 ▶ **LIQUIDS**

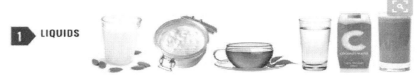

Choice of almond or another non-dairy milk, kefir, cooled herbal tea, water or coconut water, fresh-squeezed juice

2 ▶ **1 1/2 CUPS GREENS**

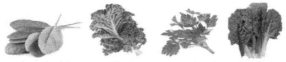

Any combination of Spinach, Kale, Parsley, Chard

3 ▶ **1 TO 1/2 CUP FRESH OR FROZEN FRUIT**

Vitamin K and potassium boost:

Extra fiber:

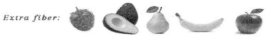

Immunity and antioxidant boost:

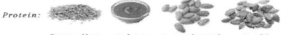

Extra omega-3s:

4 ▶ **NUTRITION BOOSTING EXTRAS**

Protein:

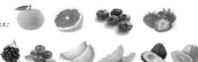

Bee pollen, nut butter, raw almonds, pumpkin seeds

Detoxing and a metabolism boost:

1 teaspoon turmeric, cinnamon or grated fresh ginger, basil, mint

Extra fiber:

2 tablespoons chia seeds or chopped dates

Omega-3s:

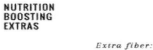

2 tablespoons raw walnuts or flax oil/seeds

5 ▶ **SWEETENERS**

1/2 teaspoon all-natural vanilla extract or agave nectar, extra banana, 1 teaspoon raw honey

Here are some recipes:

SMOOTHIE	1 CUP* FRESH GREENS	1.5 CUPS FROZEN FRUIT	PROTEIN	1 CUP LIQUID	OPTIONAL FANCY STUFF
GREEN MANGO	SPINACH OR KALE	MANGO	1/4 CUP YOGURT	WATER	1/4 CUP FRESH GINGER
GREEN PEACH	SPINACH OR KALE	PEACH	2 TBSP HEMP	COCONUT WATER	1/4 TSP GROUND CINNAMON
BANANA NUT	SPINACH OR KALE	BANANA	1/4 CUP NUTS (ANY)	MILK (ANY)	1 TBSP COCOA POWDER
PIÑA-COLADA	SPINACH OR KALE	PINEAPPLE	1 TBSP CHIA SEEDS	COCONUT WATER	1 TBSP SHREDDED COCONUT
BERRY	SPINACH OR KALE	BERRIES	2 TBSP ROLLED OATS	MILK (ANY)	1/2 BANANA
CHERRY NUT	SPINACH OR KALE	CHERRIES	2 TBSP NUT BUTTER (ANY)	MILK (ANY)	1/4 TSP VANILLA EXTRACT

More Tips for Healthy Eating:

- Limit foods from the top shelves, because they are high in fat, sugar, and salt.
- Always use fresh foods. Learn to cook and prepare your own meals.
- When choosing the food, always read the nutrition label and check the portion of fat, sugar, and salt.
- Eat fruits and vegetables every day. It would be very good if you choose five or more different colored fruits and vegetables.
- The best foods to fuel the body are whole grain bread, cereals, whole-wheat pasta, and brown rice.
- Avoid fried foods, instead choose steaming, grilling, and baking.
- Eat fish at least once a week. It contains important minerals and vitamins.
- Use very little salt or no salt at all.
- Eat slowly and enjoy your food. Always eat breakfast. Avoid alcohol.

Low-carb diet and insulin

Low-carb diets are supposed to decrease insulin levels - which can help the body to burn stored fat for energy. If the diet works correctly, your body should be in a near-constant state of fat burning, which can be an effective way to lose weight.

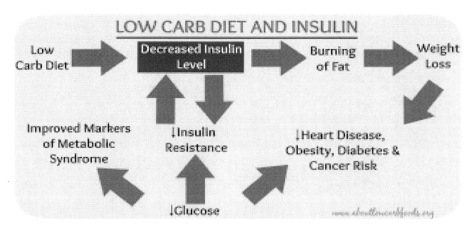

The basic idea is to eat an ultra-low carb (less than 30 gm) to induce ketosis which primes your body to burn fat while preserving muscle. Then once a week, after your weight workout, load up on a massive amount of high glycemic index carb. This will incite a large insulin spike which tells the body that there is plenty of food around, preventing the typical down regulation of metabolism seen in starvation.

Keto Diet

In this method, if you raise insulin even slightly by eating carbs 30 or more grams, it will be enough—you will seriously impair your body's ability to burn fat for the rest of the day. Worse, you may even get fatter because of the presence of another hormone, cortisol. A stress hormone, cortisol will break down fat all morning, but combined with raised insulin, it can actually cause your body to create new fat cells.

Indian Keto diet

Indian Keto diet consists of 70-80% fat, 10-15% protein, and 5-10% carbs. Salads are good but you shouldn't make that the main portion of your diet since veggies can be high in carbs. 3-4 cups of veggies are all you need on this diet.

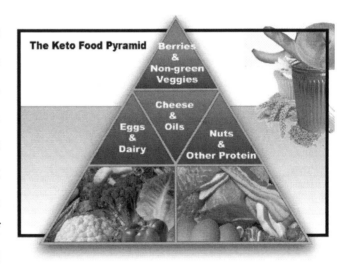

You must remember that each individual's body has a different metabolic rate so you should consult a dietitian before you go ahead with this!

If you've decided to try the ketogenic diet, you would definitely need to take some time to plan your meals. Firstly, just reflect and figure out the amount of carbohydrates you eat every day. Now decide how much you can cut them from each meal. Carbohydrates should not be more than 15% of your entire day's diet. You should plan a diet such that each meal contains just 5% carbohydrates.

To begin with, try and cut down the traditional sources of carbs. If you eat three chapatis for lunch, reduce it to two. Eat only one chapati for dinner.

Green leafy vegetables, root vegetables and fruits contain lots of vitamins and minerals and they supply very less calories to the body. They can easily supply the required amount of carbs to your body every day. Moreover, they make you feel fuller faster and for longer periods of time.

Avoid eating refined flour since it can affect your gastrointestinal system adversely and also contains lots of calories.

Stay away from aerated drinks, packaged juices and sodas as they contain lots of sugars and they will put all your efforts in vain.

If you follow quantified nutrition strictly for 4 weeks, guaranteed 8 kgs weight loss. Please, no cheating, no sugars, restrict carbs, no alcohol. It is difficult for 3 -5 days but once the body adjusts to changes it will be fine. You might feel irritated, headaches, little fever but all will go in less than 5 days. Limited black coffee/tea is allowed.

Your breakfast should consist of 3-4 eggs with yolks. You can make omelets or have them boiled, scrambled or poached. You can cook it in coconut oil, olive oil, butter or ghee if you want.

What can you eat for lunch?

1. Eggs (2-4) in any form with butter or cheese,
2. 200-300 grams meat/fish,
3. Paneer
4. Low glycemic Vegetables, butter milk or curd (full fat),
5. Dinner can be the same as lunch, skip the curd.

What snacks can you eat?

1. Fistful of cashew nuts, peanuts or 10 grams butter/cheese,
2. Vegetables: Lettuce, Jalapenos, Olives, Broccoli, Cucumber.
3. Meat: Chicken, Fish, Lamb, Bacon.
4. Fat: Paneer, Ghee, Butter, Cheese, Coconut Oil.

My Herb List

Ginger, Holi Basil, Neem, Triphala, Guggul	Diabetes
Ginger, Triphala Turmeric, Trikatu	Digestion
Amla, Chvanprash, Ginger, Tulsi, Neem, Turmeric	Immune System
Ashgandha, Ginger, Guggul, Boswellia, Neem, Shilajit, Turmeric	Joints
Chavanprash, Guggul, Triphala, Gymnema, Sylvestre, Turmeric	Weight Control
Boswellia, Shilajit, Turmeric	Back
Amla, Neem, Turmeric	Hair

How to Make Healthy Protein Bars at Home

Most of the protein bars that you can buy in the market are filled with sugar, artificial sweeteners and other not healthy components. That's why I have started to make my own Protein Bars.

Here are two great homemade protein bar recipes that I use every month: baked and unbaked versions.

Option#1 - Peanut butter Oat Protein Bar - Need Baking in Oven

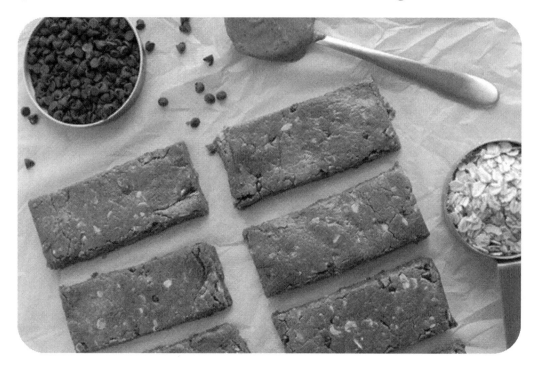

Ingredients

- 1 cup old fashioned oat, 1/2 cup flax seeds or shredded coconut- put them in the food processor for 30 seconds,
- 1 Scoop protein powder,
- 2 Tbsp chia seeds,
- 1 T cocoa powder,
- 1/2 cup peanut butter,
- 1/2 cup unsweetened almond milk or normal milk,
- 1/4 cup almond, or any other nut chopped,
- Salt to taste.

Instructions

In a large bowl, combine the oats mixer, protein powder, and chia seeds.

In a small bowl, combine the peanut butter, milk. You can add honey if you want to make it a little sweet. Microwave for 40 seconds.

Add liquid mixture into dry ingredients and stir to combine.

Add water if necessary, to make sure all dry ingredients are moistened. The mixture will be crumbly.

Put a little bit of coconut oil or olive oil into an 8x8 pan and press the mixer.

Preheat Oven at 350. Put the pan inside and set the timer for 18-20 minutes.

Your protein bars will be ready to eat after 5 minutes. Rest you can store in the refrigerator and it will easily last for approximately 2 weeks.

Option#2 – Banana Bread Protein Bar - No Backing Needed
Ingredients

- ½ cup each of - banana, dates, almonds, whey (I like the Naked Whey because it is a pure form of whey protein),
- 3 tablespoons of Sesame or Chia seeds,
- 1/2 Teaspoon salt,
- ½ teaspoon cinnamon and nutmeg,
- 1-2 tablespoon of peanut butter or vanilla extract for taste if you like.

Instructions

- Mix all these together in a mixer - it becomes a paste.
- After mixing, sprout dry coconut flakes, crushed nuts or buckwheat - this will add some extra crunch.
- Put it in the refrigerator and cut it into pieces.
- You can keep these homemade bars in the refrigerator for two weeks and they will be good.

Can you give these whey protein bars to children?

People often ask if it's healthy for children and the answer is YES. Whey is in the most infant formulas and human breast milk is 60% whey. It helps to lose weight; boost immunity and some studies have shown this helps children with asthma. It's especially good for children who don't eat well or are very active. If you are making this specifically for kids, I suggest half the amount of protein powder.

Tips to buy healthy milk

I don't own a cow, which milk should I buy and drink?

When I was little there was only one type of MILK available to us: "MILK" (Whole Milk). It means that life was easy - no energy waste in the decision making of which milk to buy and drink.

Now, the Milk has become milk, Almond milk, Soya milk, 1%/2%/skim/whole, a great number of options. When we have too many options, it leads to the paradox of choices.

Okay, now here are my tips on which Milk is better (depending on your current health and allergy condition).

A person with no intolerance (digestive) or allergy issues and is not a couch potato should drink whole, organic milk in moderation. It is good for you!

You may argue that whole milk has FAT and Cholesterol. Okay, here is a funny thing that happened in 2015.

The USDA has revised its guidelines in April 2015 to state that there is no link between cholesterol consumption and heart diseases1.

Basically, what they said is "we were wrong for the last 40 years and there is no good data available to tell that consuming cholesterol leads to having a

---

[1] http://www.cnn.com/2015/02/19/health/dietary-guidelines/

cholesterol problem". USDA did not even feel sorry for doing this to us for so many years.

Almond and coconut milk are better options. It would be better if you can try to learn to make it at home. Or at least buy an unsweetened type.

Some tips to buy milk

1. Look for the expiry date: do not buy it if it's going to expire in the next 3 weeks. These milks go bad quickly after opening the bottle.
2. Learn to read the nutrition labels: look for sugar and other ingredients. Look if it's a USDA certified organic.
3. Go for unsweetened milk: otherwise, it would lead to consuming too much sugar.
4. Once the bottle is opened: look for texture, sometimes milk goes bad way before its expiry date.
5. Choose local and organic milk if possible, or at least it would be RGBS free. If you can find grass-fed organic, then it's even better.

How much water should you drink each day for brighter skin, more energy, and less fat?

Many people do not know if they are drinking enough water. Let me give you a simple formula and tips to drink more water.

An easy little formula I like to use is to take your weight in pounds, cut it in half. So, I'm like 150 pounds. Cut that in half, 75. Make sure that's the minimum amount of water you drink per day in ounces. The minimum amount of water to drink, for me, would be 75 ounces (2.3 liters) a day. My daily intake of water is around 3 liters.

Another simple rule you can apply is: Check your urine color. If your urine is always crystal clear (& not light yellow, dark yellow or reddish), you are drinking the right quantity of water. If the color is light or dark yellow means your body is not fully hydrated.

Tips to consume more water:
1. Drink 2 glasses of water immediately after waking up (about .75 liter).
2. When you feel like snacking (emotional eating), drink a glass of water first.
3. Drink a warm small cup of water before going to bed. This strategy is helpful for losing fat and keeping you hydrated.
4. Do not replace water with coffee or tea. Drink a glass of water before drinking coffee and you can reduce the dehydration and inflammation the caffeine will create.

How to read nutrition labels?

Nutrition labels are quite confusing, even for those educated in nutrition. The information below is my notes that I refer to when I buy my food items.

Step 1- Look at the quantity

Most labels use 'per 100 gram' or 'per ounce'. Find out how you consume in one portion. If you consume 200 grams of the food, you obviously need to multiply it by 2. Some products have pre-calculated serving sizes.

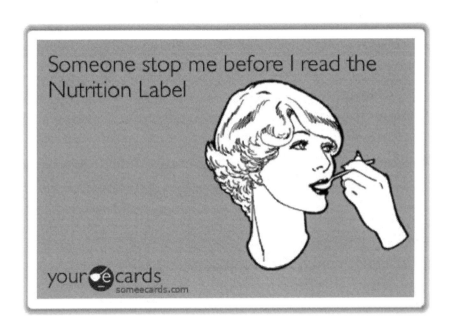

Someone stop me before I read the Nutrition Label

your ecards
someecards.com

Step 2- Look at the Macronutrients

Calories are the most important part when you look for the right food. Want to gain weight? Of course, no. Then pick one with a lot of calories per serving. If you want to lose weight you want to limit the calories per serving.

1. Protein is a great nutrient, so if food has a lot of protein, you have made a good choice. 60 grams for a 150-pound person is good enough.

2. Carbohydrates are great for energy. You can also see 'of which sugars'. Sugar should be low, one-third of the total carbohydrates or less.

3. Fats are also great for energy. However, they add up to the number of calories quickly! Look at what kind of fat it contains. Saturated and trans-fat is bad, so limit them (you should not consume more than 12-15 grams. Unsaturated fats are the good ones! When the Nutrition Facts label says a food contains "0 g" of trans fat but includes "partially hydrogenated oil" in the ingredient list, it means the food contains trans-fat, but less than 0.5 grams of trans fat per serving. So, if you eat more than one serving, you could quickly reach your daily limit of trans fat.

4. Vitamins and minerals are also great. Not all labels contain them, but if they do pick the product with the most vitamins and minerals. You can often see the percentages of daily needs for those!

Step 3- Look at the ingredients

Ingredients are ranked from common to least common. When sugar is on top of the list, most of the product contains sugar. If you are allergic to certain things this should be a habit.

Serving Size: Percent of Daily Value. This is calculated for a moderately active woman, or a fairly sedentary man, who eats 2,000 calories a day.

Sodium: The recommended daily limit for an average adult is 2,000 milligrams; too much sodium can cause high blood pressure.

Dietary Fiber: The average adult should eat between 21 and 35 grams of fiber daily, but most don't reach that level. When buying bread or cereal, look for a brand with 3 grams or more per serving.

How to Lose Weight

Losing weight is a mental game. You should be ready to sacrifice your time and efforts and love every moment you dedicate to losing your weight. If you make a habit to exercise and keep the right diet you will get fast results. First, choose an activity that you like rather than the one that is the most efficient in obtaining your goals, such as Zumba classes versus fitness boot camp.

Focus on the immediate and enjoyable aspects of your activity. For example, think about berries as a very yummy dessert. Include other immediate outside rewards, such as listening to music during exercising. That will help you reach your ultimate goals.

What is the most effective way to approach weight-loss?

The most effective approach is losing weight through diet. Before you even consider starting a formal exercise program you need to realize a trainer can work with you hard every day, but a bad diet trumps all possible progress. To be accepted as a Push Fitness client, prospects wishing to lose weight must show a willingness to improve eating habits.

I already have a balanced diet, what should I do to have the right exercises?

The ideal plan is interval training and heavy compound lifts. Intervals and heavy lifting teach your body to burn calories 'round the clock. This combination is the safest and fastest surefire way to shed fat tissue. Fad diets and quick fixes always prove temporary.

I hate cardio, what's the minimum I need to do to reach my weight-loss goals?

The answer is none. While cardiovascular exercise is important for endurance, weight-loss and heart health can be achieved without it. In the most rigorous Push Fitness strength program, cardio is contraindicated. Prospects must be evaluated for this program. They should also be prepared for intense 60-minute strength training sessions three times per week and agree to comply with all dietary regulations.

Why do we feel hungry and what we can do about it?

Some hormones crave for FAT, some crave for Protein, some for the Fiber and some for Greens. If we just eat carb-rich meals, it will increase insulin level and when insulin level comes down, we feel hungry again and crave for snacks or processed food.

The best way to deal with these hunger hormones is to have a balanced meal including FAT, Protein, Fiber, and Green. For example, your morning smoothie can be a perfect mix of Protein, Fat, Fiber, and Greens.

How to Deal with Emotional Eating

You should promise yourself that you will not do it again. It could be caused by stress, frustration, sadness. Find something to replace it, recognize it, write it down and make a habit. Close your eyes and visualize it.

Want to eat healthily? Prepare your meal on Sunday for the whole week. Want to ease your smartphone addiction? Leave it behind when you don't really need it. Visualize your goals and talk to yourself. Treat yourself but do not overindulge.

What Should You Eat Before Exercising?

Just before you exercise, the last thing you want to do is put a bunch of proteins and fats into your body. These types of fuels take a long time to digest and draw precious oxygen and energy-delivering blood into your stomach and away from your exercising muscles. They also carry a greater risk of giving you a stomachache during your exercise. But if you don't eat at all, you risk breaking down muscle and causing a great deal of stress to your body during exercise.

The ideal pre-workout meal is consumed about two hours before exercise, contains about 300-500 calories, and is composed primarily of healthy carbohydrates. If you don't have time to eat two hours before, a quick 50-100 calorie snack 5-10 minutes prior to exercise will also be effective.

Some foods that are perfect to eat before workout. Example: Greek Yogurt, Banana, Smoothie, Oatmeal, Protein bar, Apple.

Ideally, you should have some form of fuel in your system before you work out. Eating an easily digested carbohydrate an hour or so before you hit the gym ensures that you'll have enough energy in the tank to get through your program. Try fruit and yogurt or toast and peanut butter; not too much or you'll feel sluggish and heavy.

If you exercise in the morning, eating before your workout may not be an option. Many people find that they can tolerate cardio on an empty stomach but need fuel to get through a strength training session. Experiment with the types of food and the timing of your pre-workout meal to discover what works best for you.

What should you eat after a workout?

Eating after a workout is important. You need to replenish your glycogen stores and 'feed' the muscles that you've just trained. Sports nutritionists suggest that you eat a small snack consisting of protein and easily digested carbohydrates within about an hour of training and then your next meal an hour or two later.

Common post-workout nutrition 'mistakes' include eating too much (if you burn 300 calories during your workout, you don't want to be consuming a 500-calorie protein shake) and choosing less than healthy options (perhaps as a reward for working out...).

What Should You Eat While Exercising?

If you plan on exercising for less than an hour, you don't need to eat; just make sure you hydrate with small, frequent sips of water during your workout. But if you're doing something like a long run or bike ride, or maybe a couple of back-to-back fitness classes, try to eat 50-100 calories every 30 minutes, preferably from a quick carbohydrate source that is easy to carry, like a Ziplock bag of raisins, an energy bar, energy gels, or even a sports drink. The goal is not to replace every calorie that you burn, but rather to give you just enough fuel so that you can maintain a brightly burning metabolism.

Food for Cardio Days

After a cardiovascular workout (fat burning day), wait 30-45 minutes and then consume a high-quality source of protein (whole food) and vegetable-type carbohydrate. An example would be a spinach salad and some organic grilled chicken.

The reason why you'll want to wait a bit after a fat burning cardio session to eat is to ride the fat burning wave of your cardio session. However, waiting more than an hour is typically too long, and can start to slow down your metabolism because your body goes into starvation mode.

Food for Weight Training Days

After a resistance workout (muscle building day) you will need a different approach. The meal after a resistance workout is the only meal that you ever want to be absorbed rapidly. Why? Because typically, when a meal is absorbed fast because of high glycemic or simple carbs, there is a good chance your blood sugar will rise too fast, and the carbohydrates will be stored as body fat. But after a resistance workout, you've just primed the pump with an intense workout (with weights), and you have a one-hour window of opportunity to shuttle in nutrients, amino acids, glycogen, and other anabolic nutrients to repair your damaged muscles.

If you miss this one-hour window after your intense workout, the chances that your muscles will not be able to repair themselves, which makes them bigger and stronger, diminish significantly. The best post workout meal on resistance training days is whey protein and a higher glycemic (fast released, starchy) carbohydrate. You can use a banana as your carb.

For example, if your target body weight is 150lbs, you should eat about 300 calories of carbohydrate, and about half that many calories of protein. A sample post-workout meal could be chicken with brown rice, yogurt with almonds, or a protein shake with a banana.

How to keep the weight off

1. Nourish your body.

Many of us are chronically malnourished and that causes our cells to not function properly. So, add lots of superfoods and real foods, like live salad greens, green juices, super greens, spirulina, chlorella, sprouts. The key is to add these foods for medicinal purposes. Don't think of them as food, think of them as medicine. You're eating them to heal.

2. Heal your digestion.

There's a lot of studies out now that show having unfriendly bacteria in your intestines or having leaky gut can cause chronic low-grade inflammation. So, add lots of fermented foods, like sauerkraut, kimchi, nutritional yeast, probiotics, coconut kefir, coconut yoghurts and nut cheeses. Also add bone broths as they have collagen that helps heal the intestines. Again, the focus is always on adding for medicinal purposes. I usually have a couple of tablespoons of fermented veggies before each meal for example.

3. Get lots of sleep

Not having enough sleep elevates cortisol levels, which causes leptin and insulin resistance. Get lots of sleep. Also take a nap in the afternoon if you can.

4. Reduce mental stress

Mental stress, just like any other type of stress causes hormonal changes in your body. For some of us, it causes the hormonal changes that activate The FAT Programs. So, develop daily mind-body practices to heal mental stress, such as meditation, visualization, yoga and chi kung.

5. Work through emotional issues

Emotional issues can cause an elevation of stress hormones and emotional trauma can cause weight gain. So, address any emotional trauma you've had in your life.

6. Develop a detoxification lifestyle

Toxicity is a chronic stress that can cause weight gain. For starters, drink lots of water to help flush out toxins. When possible add organic produce. If you eat meat, try to make sure it's organic and grass fed, free range or wild caught. By having more organic produce and following the other suggestions above, which will also help detoxify your body, you can develop a 'detoxification lifestyle'. A detoxification lifestyle is when you're passively eliminating toxins in a gentle way, day by day, so that each day you are cleaner and healthier.

7. Address life issues

Sometimes your life is the problem. When you ignore the issues in your life that are not ideal, such as being in the wrong career, relationship or location, it causes chronic stress, which can cause your body to gain weight. Be willing to make some changes. Use visualization and affirmations to help you make the life changes that are necessary. When meditating ask for help from your intuition, higher self, invisible guides, guardian angels or God. However, you conceive the invisible support in your life, connect with it and ask it for help. Then when the time comes and the opportunity presents itself, allow yourself to take a chance if it feels right, even if it's a bit scary.

How can I build lean muscle mass on Indian diet?

Legumes (i.e., pulses) like dal and lentils (chickpeas) are plentiful in Indian diets. When combined with whole grain foods like chapatis, you get all your essential amino acids. Snacking on nuts most days will ensure you get enough protein. If you like meat, preparing meat with Indian foods will also ensure you get enough protein, plus the other benefits of a healthy Indian diet.

"I get so many vegetables every night, so I must be eating healthy."

Many Indian dishes are made by deep-frying vegetables or cooking them in excess heat. This destroys most of the vitamins and other phytonutrients, so your body won't get the benefits of these plant foods. To prevent this from happening, sauté or flash boil them. Or, if you must have your deep-fried dishes, eat raw plants by having fresh salads with your meals.

Eat avocados, nuts (like almonds, walnuts, peanuts, etc.), flaxseeds, fatty fish (like tuna, sardines, trout, etc.), olive oil. You can consider taking fish oil supplements also.

How to Eat Out Without Getting Fat

If you live in the real world, you're going to have to eat out occasionally – be it because you're traveling, meeting someone after a long time, meeting a client, or because you're working late and need to order in food – you will have to find a way to be able to eat outside food without messing up your health.

When you're eating out, the first rule is to never eat something that's completely unhealthy – this means no cake, no sugary drinks, and no white bread with processed cheese (looking at you, garlic bread). You want to have something that's composed of healthy ingredients – meats, vegetables, fruits, healthier breads and the like, even if it's cooked in an unhealthy way.

Let's take, for example, you're going to Subway, a popular chain sandwich shop. They have tons of white bread and sauces that are bad for your health, cookies that are also bad for your health, etc., But you can have a decently healthy meal there if you pick healthy ingredients.

Pick meats or paneer (cottage cheese) as the stuffing (high protein), no cheese (processed), multigrain bread, extra mustard (low calories), lots of veggies, little to none of the high-calorie sauces – chipotle sauce, southwest sauce, etc. No cookies, water is fine.

And just like that, you've had a decent meal. When you're out at a fine dining restaurant, order for eggs, salads (even though they may not be worth the money), things loaded with paneer, meats, legumes, and other high protein items. In short: ALWAYS PICK HIGH PROTEIN DISHES.

Do not consume any soft drinks, even if they are free. The price is not the money; it's your health – which is far more valuable. In fact, if you go to a restaurant often enough and the bills are high enough – they'll offer you free items on the house – usually dessert (ice cream/pastries) for everyone. Same as above, don't have it, the real price is not the money. Tell the waiter that you want your meal to be cooked in butter instead of margarine (unhealthy butter substitute) and ask him to lower the quantities of sauces.

Eat slowly and chew your food. Half of the digestion happens in your mouth. The main reason for inflammation is that people do not chew their food properly.

This prevents you from overeating and makes you more likely to get full on a lower quantity of food. Chew your food – aids digestion. If you don't like the taste of something, don't eat it. The "if you ordered it, you have to eat it" is something parents tell children to get them to order sensible dishes – you are an adult. Why would you eat something that's unhealthy when you don't even enjoy the experience? It makes no sense. If you can pay more and make your dish healthier – do it. This means paying to substitute the white bread for the brown/multigrain bread, oil for butter, etc. Extra protein is always worth paying extra for.

SUPPLEMENTATION

There are N numbers of supplements available in the market these days, be it L-Carnitine, HMB, CLA, NO products and so on and if you start buying them all, you'll probably have no money left in your pocket. See these products work, they have years of solid research backing up their claims, but there are two things to consider: 1. It's just 5% of your entire 100% and 2. For this mere 5%, it costs a BOMB! Who has the money for this idiotic advantage of 5%, right? Instead give 100% in your diet and training efforts.

Here, I'll only cover the most basic and most essential supplements.

Protein

Not going to discuss this! You need this no matter how good your diet is, don't fall for expensive isolates though, blends are good too.

How much? 1.6-1.8 gm per kg of lean body weight is decent.

Creatine

It gives you more energy to lift! Quite literally!

When lifting heavy weights, your body primarily uses ATP (Adenosine triphosphate) and CP (Creatine phosphate) stores, however these are very limited, and you cannot push any further until the body makes more ATP from glycogen again. Also, most of this ATP actually exists in the body in the form of ADP (adenosine di-phosphate). When Creatine monohydrate is introduced in the body, it binds to the phosphorus inside the body and exists as Creatine phosphate. Now this Creatine phosphate during heavy workouts gives its phosphate to ADP to form ATP, this happens much faster than glycogen to ATP conversion, thereby there's a notable increase in your strength. Creatine is one of the most well researched supplements available in the market and should be used by anyone who lifts weight.

Now there's a common myth among the bodybuilding community, that Creatine retains water. So, let's address that. First of all, what do you mean by water retention? The water is stored in your muscle cells as well as outside of your muscle cells under the skin.

This extracellular water stored under the skin is called Water Retention. It's a defense mechanism employed by the body to keep you hydrated all the time. Now Creatine draws water directly into the muscles and not into the extracellular skin, which is a good thing. Tell this to the experts and they'll be rolling their eyes now. Most of the time, these people stop drinking water all together and stop consuming sodium as well. Now sodium is one major electrolyte that helps in regulation of water in the body. So, when the body detects low levels of sodium and water, the hormone aldosterone is triggered, which further as a part of the body's defense mechanism tries to hang onto the water, thereby causing water retention intracellular as well as extracellular. And people thought it was due to Creatine.

For creatine you can go with any brand. Here is a link on amazon you can use - https://www.amazon.com/shop/agilefitness360

BCAA (Branched Chain Amino Acids)

You don't really need it if you have enough protein intake which has a complete amino acid profile. BCAA acids are basically essential amino acids which are synthesized in the body, namely leucine, isoleucine and valine along with many other amino acids. However, what makes these BCAA's more important is the role they play. These amino acids are being used by the body for energy when you're lifting heavy weights. And if the body starts making these amino acids it will not manufacture other amino acids at the same speed. And we know that all the amino acids are required for building proteins which are nothing but chains of amino acids. It is always a good idea to supplement these essential amino acids, thereby giving the body enough time to make all other amino acids, further leading to more muscle protein synthesis. However, if your protein intake for the day is sufficient, then you do not need to supplement with BCAA.

Zinc Magnesium

ZMA or Zinc Magnesium Aspartate is a mineral supplement that is a combination of Zinc Aspartate, Magnesium Aspartate and Vitamin B6. The reason ZMA has become popular amongst athletes and people who do resistance training is because it supplements mainly with zinc and magnesium which is studied to be deficient in people who train.

Zinc has been proven to be vital for the activity of more than 300 enzymes. Those enzymes aid in macronutrient metabolism and cell replication, which as we know are key biochemical functions that correspond to recovery and growth. Zinc has shown to have positive effects on anabolic hormone profile, particularly testosterone. It increases free serum testosterone levels which is particularly important in older men as their testosterone levels start to decline with age.

Micronutrients

Your Multivitamin/multimineral tabs. They are not very expensive, and it's a good idea to take them. You may not realize this but if your diet doesn't have chromium in it, you will suffer poor metabolism. How?

Let me explain, even though chromium is required in micrograms, it is an essential cofactor for proper functioning of your hormone insulin. And you know how important insulin is. This is just one example showing how important these micronutrients in your body can be. There are more than 26 such vitamins and minerals that are required for optimum health by your body every day. Unfortunately, there is no single food that will provide you the full spectrum, hence supplementation becomes all the more essential. Multivitamins and minerals tablets can do that for you.

Having a balanced diet can take care of most of the micronutrients however supplementation of the following is always beneficial and is even recommended:

Vitamin C, and for vegetarians - Vitamin–B (thiamin, riboflavin, niacin, and so on).

Don't forget fish oil capsules or flaxseed oil for omega-3 and omega-6 fatty acids. Remember they are required by your brain. Similarly, garlic is a very beneficial herb.

The list goes on; I'd suggest sticking with the basics. Try to explore more herbs and check out their benefits, a fish oil capsule will cost you more but flax seeds you can get for 140rs/kg in the market.

1. Insulin

Insulin has always been propagated as the muscle building hormone and even as the fat storing hormone. Truth is, it does both and you don't need to fret much about it. It's a hormone that helps you stay stable, by keeping your blood glucose levels stable when it tends to rise due to incoming carb intake. It "opens up" the cells to take the incoming glucose in.

Insulin is a hormone made by the pancreas that allows your body to use sugar (glucose) from carbohydrates in the food that you eat for energy or to store glucose for future use. Insulin helps keep your blood sugar level from getting too high (hyperglycemia) or too low (hypoglycemia).

The cells in your body need sugar for energy. However, sugar cannot go into most of your cells directly. After you eat food and your blood sugar level rises, cells in your pancreas (known as beta cells) are signaled to release insulin into your bloodstream. Insulin then attaches to and signals cells to absorb sugar from the bloodstream. Insulin is often described as a "key," which unlocks the cell to allow sugar to enter the cell and be used for energy.

2. Glucagon

We discussed how insulin helps keep the blood glucose level stable by helping the body take in the excess glucose. Glucagon does the exact opposite by helping the blood glucose remain stable by bringing in supply of glucose when blood glucose is low, by breaking down the stored glycogen in the liver. So, insulin and glucagon are interlinked, and it's no surprise that both of them are produced in the pancreas itself.

3. Testosterone

Now testosterone is the primary male hormone which gives men their "male" characteristic, from voice to facial hair. It helps maintain proper health in men and also helps to build muscles. Now testosterone is a male hormone, but it doesn't mean that women don't produce it. Even women produce it, but much less than men. Women are more sensitive to this hormone. A healthy testosterone level is important for you for proper muscle gain and fat loss. So, make sure your micronutrients are on point and that you are not a hypocaloric diet for long. (Note – there is a difference between calorie deficit and hypocaloric. Hypocaloric diet here means severe deficit for a long time.) The best testosterone booster in nature is lifting heavy weights. If you lift weights, your testosterone production gets better, thereby aiding in muscle build up and strength gains (in women, "toning" is essentially muscle build up itself, along with fat loss. Lifting weights will help you do that instead of aerobics).

4. Estrogen

Estrogen is the female counterpart of testosterone. It makes a woman, a woman. It is responsible for the development and regulation of the female reproductive system and secondary sex characteristics. Now there are several different types of estrogen too, but that is beyond the scope of this book

for now. One thing to remember here is, it is a very important hormone for women. And lifting weights will NOT bring it down to affect your health. Another concern among men is about the increase of estrogen in their bodies due to soya consumption. That won't happen unless you eat 1 kilo raw soya everyday continuously for months at a stretch. So there's nothing to worry about.

5. Leptin

Leptin is a very important hormone in your body that's essential for fat loss. It is like your fuel indicator that signals your brain about the availability of food and based on that your brain holds on to your body's fat stores or goes easy on them to release them for use. That's directly related to metabolic adaptation (how your body controls and varies your metabolism). This hormone goes

down when you are on a caloric deficit for too long, and the effect is more if carbs are omitted from the diet. This is the reason why a refeed helps. A well-timed and well-placed refeed can help you lose more by raising your leptin levels after a short dieting phase.

6. Cortisol

In the fitness community, cortisol is seen as the villain. Truth is, it is neutral. Depends on how it functions and the scenario it functions in. It is a catabolic hormone that helps in the metabolism of fat, protein and carbohydrate – all three. So even your fat loss is dependent on cortisol. However, excess amounts of cortisol for extended time periods is bad as it can metabolize your muscle mass too. Cortisol is released in response to stress and low blood glucose concentration.

How to convince your significant other to follow a Healthy Lifestyle?

This seems to be a very common issue among couples nowadays. The common stories are "whenever we go out, she orders junk and I order things like eggs/chicken and she forces me to taste her food and we end up hogging it ". See, I understand the emotion behind 'Opposite attracts" but when it comes to food habits in a relationship, couples have to find a common ground somewhere to keep it going, because food is the most common thing which you will be sharing almost daily and it is the only time where you will be actually spending time together because anyway rest of the day you are busy in work, phone, meetings, commute, etc. And your food habits will pass on to your kids, and your kid will become the same and imagine feeding junk to your kid in 2020.

How to convince?

Get a blood test done, together. Yes, find some couple packages and get a test done together. Reports will eventually force them to adopt a healthy lifestyle.

Start doing challenges together. There are many apps which record your steps/run count and workout timings. You can ask them to complete 3k steps daily for starters and then slowly reach to 10k. Fixing food habits only won't help; you will have to start physical activity too.

Follow your own diet and workout on a daily basis and completely. When results are achieved, share them, "I lose 2 inch, or 10 pounds and I feel great and energetic". Take it easy and take it slow. It can take easily up to 3 to 12 months to convince them about a healthy lifestyle and workouts.

SECTION 4

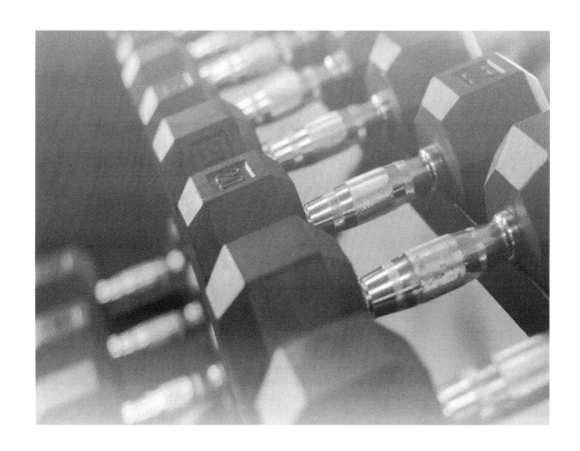

HUMAN LONGEVITY

AND BIO HACK

LONGEVITY

"To live a healthy and long life it is important to learn about the top cause of death".

The Center for Disease Control (CDC) puts together a report each year on all the registered deaths in the United States. The most recent data comes from 2013, which saw a total of 2.6M Americans pass away, with an average life expectancy of 78.8 years. The top ten leading causes of death cover 74% of all deaths in the nation, with the top three alone accounting for 52%.

The leading causes of death are the following:

1. Heart disease: 611,105 (23.5%)

2. Cancer: 584,881 (22.5%)

3. Chronic lower respiratory diseases: 149,205 (5.7%)

4. Accidents: 130,557 (5.0%)

5. Stroke: 128,978 (5.0%)

6. Alzheimer's disease: 84,767 (3.3%)

7. Diabetes: 75,578 (2.9%)

8. Influenza and pneumonia: 56,979 (2.2%)

9. Kidney diseases: 47,112 (1.8%)

10. Suicide: 41,149 (1.6%)

Risk factors and preventative steps

1. Heart disease: Lowering blood pressure and cholesterol can significantly lower heart disease risk as well as regular exercise. Avoid excessive alcohol use. Quit smoking.

2. Cancer: Lung cancer is the leading cancer. Quit smoking would solve a significant portion of these smoking-related cancers. Avoid excessive alcohol use. For skin cancer, avoid excessive direct sun exposure and wear sunscreen. More generally, many cases of cancer can be linked to being overweight, obese, or inactive.

3. Chronic lower respiratory diseases: Largely caused by smoking, so quit smoking. Also avoid air pollutants at home and in the workplace.

4. Accidents: Accidents are not only a top killer, but in fact the #1 leading cause of death for Americans under 44. Auto related accidents are the top category. Nearly 1/3 of traffic-related deaths are caused by being alcohol-impaired. Avoid driving while intoxicated.

5. Stroke: High blood pressure, high cholesterol, and smoking are major risk factors for stroke. Limit alcohol.

6. Alzheimer's disease: While the exact cause of Alzheimer's disease remains unknown, it has been linked to cardiovascular disease. Therefore, reducing cardiovascular disease risk factors are helpful, including lowering blood pressure and cholesterol, exercising regularly, avoiding excessive alcohol usage, and quitting smoking.

7. Diabetes: Type 2 diabetes risk can be reduced by avoiding obesity and getting regular exercise.

8. Influenza and pneumonia: Get a flu shot every year to fight off seasonal influenza. Do not smoke. Avoid obesity and get regular exercise to better fend off all viruses.

9. Kidney diseases: Limit alcohol, quit smoking, avoid obesity.

10. Suicide: Avoid depression and substance abuse.

Define Your Health KPIs

Here are top six Health KPIs to achieve and maintain to give you the best chances of reducing the risk of the majority of top 10 leading causes of death.

1.BMI < 25

A person's Body Mass Index (BMI) is their weight (in kilograms) divided by the square of their height in meters (easily calculated through many online BMI calculators). BMI guidelines state the following healthy ranges:

< 25: Healthy
25 - 29.9: Overweight
>30: Obese
More than 69% of adult Americans are currently overweight or obese

and 35% of adult Americans are obese, putting them at significant risk for

many of the top killers in America.

To achieve a healthy BMI, it's important to devote to losing the appropriate

amount of weight necessary to get there.

2. Physical activity of 150 minutes of moderate-intensity OR 75 minutes of vigorous-intensity per week

Moderate-intensity physical activity includes brisk walking, slow biking, yoga, tennis and golf.

Vigorous-intensity physical activity includes running, swimming, fast biking, competitive sports, singles tennis, etc.

3. Limit alcohol to one serving for women or two servings for men per day

Excessive alcohol consumption is also a key risk factor for several of the leading causes of death. It's thus important to ensure that you limit your consumption to moderate alcohol consumption per day, as defined by the Dietary Guidelines for Americans, which is 1 serving for women per day and 2 servings for men per day. A drink serving is defined as 12 ounces of beer, 5 ounces of wine, or 1.5 ounces of liquor.

4. Total cholesterol < 200 mg/dL, LDL < 130 mg/dL, HDL > 40 mg/dL, triglycerides < 150 mg/dL

Cholesterol is a waxy substance that travels through your blood to various cells, produced primarily by your liver. As discussed above, high cholesterol has been shown to be a major risk factor in a variety of the leading causes of death. Cholesterol levels are measured by measuring the levels of lipoproteins, LDL and HDL, that carry cholesterol throughout the body. To get your cholesterol measured, request a lipoprotein panel blood test from your doctor.

When you get your lipoprotein panel blood test results, you'll get back 4 measures, each of which have the following healthy ranges:

Total Cholesterol < 200 mg/dL

LDL < 140 mg/dL

HDL > 40 mg/dL

Triglycerides < 150 mg/dL

Reducing cholesterol is typically achieved through increasing your physical activity, reducing your weight, improving your diet, and prescription drugs.

5. Blood pressure < 120/80 mmHg

Blood pressure is the force of the blood pushing against the walls of the arteries. Each time the heart beats (about 60-70 times a minute at rest), it pumps out blood into the arteries. Your blood pressure is at its highest when the heart beats, while pumping the blood. This is called systolic pressure. When the heart is at rest, between beats, your blood pressure falls. This is the diastolic pressure. Blood pressure is measured by these two numbers, the systolic and diastolic pressures, written one above the other, such as 120/80 mmHg. It's easily tested at your doctor's office with a simple blood pressure monitor.

An ideal blood pressure is < 120/80 mmHg.

Reducing blood pressure is typically achieved through reducing your weight, increasing physical activity, reducing alcohol consumption, reducing sodium, as well as other potential diet changes.

6. Fasting blood sugar < 100 mg/dL

While type 2 diabetes risk factors are largely reduced through achieving the other measures shown here (BMI, exercise guidelines), if you have a history of diabetes in your family, it may make sense to independently test for the risk through periodic fasting blood sugar tests. You simply fast for 8 hours and then get your blood drawn.

Fasting blood sugar guidelines state the following healthy ranges:

- < 100 mg/dL: Healthy
- 100 - 125 mg/dL: Pre-diabetes

- 125 mg/dL: Diabetes (when measured in 2 consecutive tests)

More than 35% of adult Americans have pre-diabetes, putting them at significant risk for developing type 2 diabetes, heart disease, and stroke.

Reducing fasting blood sugar is typically achieved through reducing your weight, increasing physical activity, and improving your diet (noticing a pattern yet?).

Essential Habits to Enhance Longevity

1. DIET AND EXERCISE:

Eat mostly plants, most of the time.

That means fruits, vegetables, beans and lentils, nuts and seeds, and whole grains. Avoid eating fast or fried foods, sweets and sugary beverages, and red and processed meats (like cold cuts) as much as possible.

Avoid processed and packaged food.

Even the healthy stuff that is full of agave syrup and vegetable oil in disguise.

Eat legumes.

Legumes are rich in plant protein, vitamins, minerals, appetite-satiating and gut-supporting fiber, and slow-burning carbohydrates that do not cause a large amount of glycemic variability. You may need some gut fixing first to handle.

Incorporate low-level physical activity throughout the day

Centenarians in the Blue Zones tend to lead very active lives, yet rarely set foot in a gym or Ironman start line.

Low risk alcohol intake

If you drink any alcohol, keep the recommended limits in mind: one drink per day max for women, two drinks per day max for men. Consuming wine with or before a meal can improves the absorption of the artery-scrubbing flavonoid antioxidants in the wine.

Restrict Calories (CR)

Long-term CR has been associated in multiple studies with better weight management and slowed aging, as well as a reduced risk of diseases related to metabolic health, such as type 2 diabetes, heart disease, and cancer.

2.Lifestyle and Spirit:

One of my favorite practices that my family and I participate in each morning is gratitude journaling. We start off each day by opening our journals and discussing three questions: What am I grateful for today? What truth did I discover in today's scripture reading? Who can I pray, help, or serve today?

When you introduce conscious, mindful gratitude into your day, positivity will begin to pour into your life—along with all the other scientifically proven physical, mental, and spiritual benefits of gratitude.

Here are 6 more lifestyle and spiritual tips to enhance longevity.

1. Don't smoke - that includes secondhand smoke and air pollution. Be ruthlessly cognizant of air quality.

2. Prioritize social engagement - Even if it means occasionally staying out past your bedtime or eating late at night, pros of being with people outweighs the cons of the possible disruptions to your circadian rhythm.

3. Possess a Strong Life Purpose - An eleven-year NIH-funded study found those who expressed a clear purpose for their life lived longer than those who did not, and those with purpose also stayed immersed in activities and communities involved in fulfilling that purpose.

4. Have Low Amounts of Stress - Chronic stress leads to inflammation and serves as the foundation for nearly every age-related disease.

5. Engage in a Spiritual Discipline or Religion or Believe in a Higher Power - All but 5 of the 263 centenarians in Blue Zones belong to some faith-based community.

6. Remain Reproductively Useful- the more consistently you can send your body and brain the message that you are still a valuable, contributing member of society, particularly when it comes to the propagation of your species, the longer nature will want to keep you around.

Anti-Aging Tips from Experts

I have some tips from some of my favorite fitness and longevity enthusiasts. They each contributed their non-negotiables for staying young.

Tip #1: Eat Real Food (Charles Eugster)

Variety is key. He avoids sugar and eats lots of meat, especially fat. Fat! Piles of fat. Yet, while in a supermarket he was perplexed to find yogurt with zero fat. Can you imagine a hunter-gatherer enjoying a low-fat yogurt?

Tip #2: Learn New Stuff (Laird Hamilton)

Laird's garage is chock-full of unique toys that Laird has invented to attack ocean waves in new ways. It is also packed with skis, snowboards, Jet Skis, foil boards, balance-training devices, and all manner of different tools to force his brain and muscles to maintain neurons and build new ones.

Tip #3: Lift, Move, Sprint (Mark Sisson)

Rather than engaging in long, slow chronic cardio, he instead does short, fast, all-out sprint workouts at least once a week, all year long. He doesn't overdo these and recommends performing such workouts (ultimate frisbee, high-intensity treadmill intervals, or hard uphill cycling) once every seven to ten days.

Tip #4: Do Epic Things (Don Wildman)

Don not only performed this epic workout up until his death but also went mountain biking on difficult trails for miles every single day and enjoyed stand-up paddle boarding, big-wave surfing, and even helicopter snowboarding.

Tip #5: Train Eccentrically (Art De Vany)

The ripped, eighty-year-old Art De Vany, one of the founders of the ancestral fitness movement, gets away with extremely short weight-training episodes of just fifteen minutes per day by using an exercise strategy called "eccentric training." Eccentric training refers to the lengthening or lowering portion of a lift, during which the muscle tends to become more stressed and stimulated compared to the concentric, positive, lifting phase of an exercise.

Tip #6: Stay Supple (Olga Kotelko)

Olga didn't beat up her body without going out of her way to recover and stay supple. Book a weekly or monthly massage or do short, daily foam-rolling routines.

Tip# 7: Black Coffee and Vitamin D (Sanjeev Chopra)

Drink coffee- switch between caffeinated and decaf. Take vitamin D, Eat Nuts - Brazil nuts, almonds. Meditate once a day. If you do not have time, then do it twice a day.

How to Deal with Frequent Cold or Flu Problem

No one likes catching the cold or flu. But if it's cold outside we should know some tricks to conquer it to be more comfortable and energetic.

Here are my tips for that:

- Rest
- No processed sugar - no caffeine
- Wash hands frequently and properly
- Drink warm water
- Gargle with saltwater
- Clean up your nose using saltwater
- Take shower with hot water
- Have tea with lemon and honey
- Consume Vitamin C
- Try Turmeric and sugar kapa haka

- Do Yoga
- Do not blow your nose hard- instead clean with water or wet clothes

How to fix sleep issues naturally?

1. Exercise in the morning. Late Evening workout interferes with sleep and will keep you awake till late at night.

2. Spend 15 minutes in the sunlight. I prefer going out early in the morning when the sunlight is there but is not very shiny yet.

3. Have a light dinner. If you expect a heavy dinner (party, traveling) then eat early by 7:30 pm.

4. Have the evening wind up ritual.

5. Switch off all electronic devices at least 1 hour before sleep.

6. Brush and floss. A clean month really helps in a good night sleep and it is a healthy lifestyle.

7. Reading a book before bed is great.

8. Drink a small glass of warm water or warm turmeric milk before bed

9. Give yourself time to fall asleep - do not worry if you are awake for 1 hour and could not sleep. The key is to stay lying in bed. Do some deep and slow belly breathing.

10. Try to feel gratefulness. Remember all the good things you have in life (you are alive, have a good job, family, friends.) – feel real gratitude and be thankful to God (or whatever you believe in).

11. Prepare a good environment. Remove phone or TV from the room. The world will be there when you wake up. TRUST ME!

12. Keep the room temperature low - I recommend 65 to 67 F.

13. Make the room completely dark and quiet. Switch off all the lights. Use a curtain if the light is coming from outside through the window.

14. Wear comfortable/loose clothes.

15. Herbs/Supplement. If you are currently stressed and find it hard to sleep supplements like magnesium and melatonin are great to fix the sleep problem.

16. Drink banana tea. Wash cut in half organic banana, put it in hot water and drink.

17. Drink Chamomile Tea before bed. Make the tea and consume it 30 minutes before sleep.

18. Take a hot bath with EPSOM Salt. Put a cup of salt in the bathtub with hot water and sit in it for 15-20 minutes. This will provide magnesium and melatonin to your body and make you sleep better.

19. Don't consume caffeine after 2 PM.

20. If you plan to drink, then stop drinking alcohol for 3 hours before bedtime. Keep in mind that bedtime should not shift much from your regular sleeping window. So, plan accordingly.

21. Don't use sugar after dinner.

22. Buy blue light blocking glasses and use them when working on computer/phone/iPad after 7 pm.

23. Tell yourself that you are going to sleep like a kid. Do positive affirmation. Our mind believes in what we tell it. If you say I have had a sleep problem from the last decade and I can't sleep - the mind will believe in it. And if you say, I am going to sleep like a baby in the next 15 minutes for the next 8 hours - the mind will start to believe in it. Just try it!

How to know your body has recovered from mental and physical stress?

How do you know if you have recovered from mental/physical stress and are ready to workout, ready to run, or ready to start something new?

When I wake up in the morning, I want to feel that my body is truly ready to workout rather than just assuming it. Because if my body is not ready to work out after a few days I will end up with the muscle strain, an infection or just feeling worn-out.

However, to be fit and make progress, you have to go outside your recovery comfort zone, but you also have to know a good method for you to identify exactly how far outside that comfort zone you have gone.

Let's first understand what overtraining is and how it can affect your body and health.

Overtraining is an accumulation of training and/or non-training stress resulting in a long-term decrease in performance capacity with or without related physiological and psychological signs and symptoms of overtraining in which restoration of performance capacity may take from several weeks to several months.

Your body hits multiple stages before it goes to an overtraining state where you see the diminishing returns.

The first state is alarm. It is the first stage where your body, in response to stress, goes into overdrive in anti-stress mode, also known as the "fight or flight" response. This is the state that most athletes spend a great majority of the time. But they also know how to recover quickly.

The next states are exhaustion and failure and at these points, there is a total failure of your adrenal glands to respond to stress - which means you move into an overtraining state.

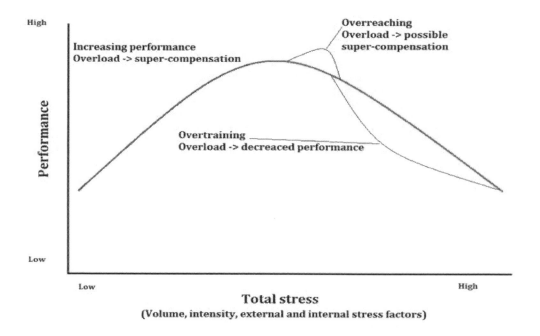

Performance vs. Total stress (Volume, intensity, external and internal stress factors)

- Increasing performance Overload -> super-compensation
- Overreaching Overload -> possible super-compensation
- Overtraining Overload -> decreaced performance

So, now you know the importance of recovery. It's time to learn how to know if your body is truly recovered and here are nine simple ways:

1. Trouble having a good sleep: Having trouble getting to sleep at night, tossing and turning throughout the night, waking up much earlier than usual (early adrenal fatigue stages) or much later than usual (later adrenal fatigue stages) can all be signs of inadequate recovery.

2. Hydration: Urine color: You can simply pay attention to your urine color-- look for pale to slightly yellow color (unless you've been taking a multivitamin, which tends to make your urine bright yellow).

3. Appetite: If you're not getting hungry anymore, it can be a sign that you're under-recovered. Your appetite typically decreases with under-recovery, high training load, and fatigue, which can create yet another vicious cycle.

4. Resting heart rate: Measure your resting heart rate and compare it with other normal days when you are not training. If you see a big variation it means your recovery is not complete.

5. Muscle soreness: Persistent muscle soreness is one sign of overreaching and overtraining. Muscle soreness should go away within 48 hours even if you had a killing leg workout session (assuming your diet is right).

6. Energy level: The trick is to be able to distinguish between days when you are truly recovered but may just feel tired versus days when your tiredness indicates a true need to rest. The best way is by writing it down and keeping a track.

7. Sudden weight loss: An acute body mass loss of 2% or greater (meaning you wake up one day and you simply weigh a lot less) can adversely affect cognitive and physical performance. So regular monitoring of pre-breakfast body mass can aid in optimizing fluid and energy balance, lead to more efficient recovery and potentially improve performance.

8. Previous day(s) performance: If your performance drops in a row for a couple of days compared to what you could do the week or month prior is a good indicator of under-recovery. Of course, you can't set a personal record every time you step into a gym so underperformance should be expected in a properly constructed training plan. But prolonged underperformance is a reliable indicator of subpar recovery.

9. I do not know the ninth way. It is up to you to decide what you can do to help you recover quickly. It could be related to your thoughts, mood, diet, life problems, working pressure, etc. Identify one good way that will help you get out of stress quickly and be healthy all the time.

Recovery: should you use ice or heat on an injury or pain?

It can sometimes be confusing whether to use heat or cold when treating sore muscles or an injury. My mother was having chronic shoulder pain for quite some time and then last week she twisted her ankle when we went for a hike. I wanted to make sure that we use the right compression method, so I did my research and here is my learning that explains when to use heat when to use cold, when not to use any of these and why.

(Note: I am not playing as a doctor, so take these facts as a grain of salt).

How heat and cold compression affect body:

- Heat: brings more blood to the area where it is applied, reduces joint stiffness and muscle cramps which makes it useful when muscles are tight.
- Cold: relieves pain by numbing the affected area, reduces swelling and inflammation and reduces bleeding.

Examples of when to use what?

- Heat: Heat is helpful for muscles, chronic pain, and to reduce stress. Heat is great for sore muscles, joint pain and for soothing the nervous system and the mind, which are typical of chronic injuries. Stress and fear are major factors in many chronic pain problems.

Example: back pain, shoulder pain or neck pain.

- Cold: Ice is the recommended treatment for acute injuries or injuries that show signs of inflammation and swelling. Cold numbs the affected area, which can reduce pain and tenderness.

Examples: a freshly pulled muscle or a new case of IT band syndrome.

What is the right timing?

- Ice is most effective when it is applied early and often for the first 48 hours. Heat Should NOT be used for the first 48 hours following an injury.

- Athletes with chronic injuries should apply heat before exercise to increase flexibility and to stimulate blood flow to the area. After exercise, ice is the best choice for a chronic injury because it discourages the onset of swelling and pain.
- Do not use ice or heat longer than 20 minutes at a time. Be sure the area goes numb when ice is applied and then make sure the skin returns completely back to normal before reapplying.
- Heat and inflammation are a particularly bad combination. If you add heat to a fresh injury it may get worse.

Summary: Remember this: Ice is for injuries, and heat is for muscles.

Best stretching and rehab sequence for pain/stiffness:

DO	DON'T
1. Start with slow dynamic stretches (neck, shoulders, legs)	1. No over stretch. make progress slowly
2. Isometric stretching	2. Do not be impatient. It's a 6-month game, and you will be better for sure.
3. Static stretching (hamstring, glutes)	3. Do not get scared by what google search or even your doc says. You can take control and become stronger and more flexible than even before.
4. Hyperbolic (optional- if want more flexibility)	
5. Do it 2x each day.	

Productivity: How to Have a Highly Productive Day?

This is a simple guide on how you can have a very productive day.

STEP 1: Make a TO – DO list

This has to be done the day before. Preferably right before you sleep. It's hard to be productive when you don't know what you want to get done.

Also, a to-do list reminds you that there are things you need to get done before you can rest. Don't make it on a phone – use a physical pen and paper. Having to check your phone again and again can be distracting for many.

STEP 2: Sleep Well and Wake up naturally.

"IF I HAD 8 HOURS TO CHOP DOWN A TREE, I WOULD SPEND 6 OF THOSE HOURS SHARPENING MY AXE." – ABRAHAM LINCOLN

Your brain is the axe.

Why would you spend 18 hours a day working hard with a blunt axe? It doesn't make sense. Remember, a well-rested mind is a sharp, focused mind. Your attention span will be longer, you'll process things faster, and you will feel better while you're at it. Ideally, you want to wake up naturally without an alarm. Go to bed early if you have to.

STEP 3: Coffee, Workout and Cold Shower

Immediately after waking up, you want to have a coffee (no sugar). Caffeine is a powerful drug – most of its potential is wasted.

We will then do a full body stretch, from the neck to the calves. You also want to add in 10 squats, 10 pushups and 10 pullups (if you have a pull-up bar) to help get the blood flowing. Once we're done, we're going to take a cold shower. A cold shower wakes you up, makes you alert, and gets the blood flowing.

STEP 4: Meditate and Hydrate

We'll start with meditation, which we will do for 20 minutes. By now you should have drunk ~1 liter of water.

STEP 5: Getting Started with The Small Tasks

Note that we're going to be skipping breakfast for now. We will quickly finish off the small things on our to-do list. Anything that takes less than 10 minutes to finish gets done here. Around 1.5 to 2 hours have passed since you woke up.

STEP 6: 2 Hours in The Zone

You want to start getting some real work done. Put your phone on silent, turn off the noise and get to work. You should have an intense amount of focus now – use that to get the tasks that require the highest amount of attention to detail done. Your brain is extremely alert, and you won't be missing subtle things. If you're a student, you want to pick a technical subject here to study.

Don't break your attention with anything – no email checking, no texting, no answering random phone calls. Don't break the flow. The momentum will help you get things done 2x better than normal.

STEP 7: Breakfast

Okay, so you've done quite a bit in those 2 hours (likely done more already than most people get done in their entire day), and you're feeling a bit sluggish.

We're going to eat filling, high-calorie items here, that don't take a lot of time/effort to prepare:

Eggs fried in butter: Makes a great breakfast, provides a lot of protein, and enough fat to help digest everything better.

Dried Fruits: Some almonds, cashews, walnuts, dates, and raisins. Excellent sources of minerals and vitamins and will provide you with the energy you need to charge through the day.

The advantage of a high-calorie breakfast is that it'll keep you full for the next "on" block, and since we're largely avoided high carb foods (such as cereal, parathas, donuts, and pastries) – we won't have the post-lunch slump that plagues corporate ~~slaves~~ employees around the world. You can listen to some music around this time and respond to any urgent phone calls you may have received.

STEP 8: 4 Hours in The Zone

The process is similar to before, but this time we'll work for 4 hours. It has been my experience that this is the best time for creative tasks – most of my articles are written during this time. Students should use this time to study subjects that involve lots of intellect and creativity. Also, same as before – no distractions, no answering phone calls, no checking emails.

STEP 9: Lunch

We will have a heavy lunch (but not too heavy). High to moderate protein is a must. You can have your carbs here – a large part of the day is already done.

Meats, rice, potatoes, grains, vegetables, legumes. No sugar drinks though – only water (you can have fruit juices without added sugars here).

Some people like to take power naps around this time, but I have not found them useful. You can take a small post-lunch walk though, 10 – 15 minutes.

STEP 10: 2 Hours in The Zone

Same as above. This part of time is best suited for dull, boring work that you have to power through. We've already done enough through the day, and now we'll go all out. You'll notice that this part is downright tedious, and you don't have the same amount of focus, attention, or creativity as you did earlier. Nevertheless, the day is coming to an end, and we're just going the extra mile.

STEP 11: Workout

Notice we didn't do a workout in the morning. This is intentional. If you're going to be working out in the morning, you'll have some amount of exhaustion throughout the day. This is not ideal for productivity. Evening workouts make more sense – after you've hit most of your targets for the day. Start with some warmup, do some cardio, lift weights. All in, this takes around 1.5 – 2 hours, depending upon your speed and intensity. Come back home and take another cold shower.

STEP 12: Dinner, Read, Relax, Sleep

So the day is almost over, we've meditated, we've eaten healthy, we've put in ~8 hours of highly productive effort, we've exercised our body – today was a good day. Now you can relax – read a book or two, listen to some music, browse the internet – whatever you like. Have a light (or heavy, depending on your mood) dinner – high to moderate protein as usual.

It has almost been 15 – 16 hours since we woke up. We'll now go to bed, pleasantly making a note of how much we've accomplished today.

Some other Pointers

1. Do not consume any alcohol throughout the day and the day before.
2. Make sure that the dinner you have the day before does not leave you bloated in the morning.

3. Avoid distractions and unnecessary screen time – no watching TV, YouTube videos or anything else that breaks the "flow" of the day.

How to stay in shape while travelling?

We are creatures of habit & routines. While doing our daily job, we can stick to a routine easily. For example, we wake up around the same time, eat all meals at the same time, work out at the same time, go to sleep at the same time, etc. However, during travelling we can't stick to our daily routines. This happened to me recently. I have tried different things and finally created a specific action plan which was very successful. You can try this during your next trip, whether it's for a week or month(s).

- Keep Exercise on the Priority list. You can have different activities, but you should also find time for exercising. Add it to your calendar, set up an email reminder, do whatever it takes. Do it constantly, it doesn't matter if you wake up early or work late at night.
- Make reasonable choices for your meals. Take the time to evaluate the menu. Select foods that are steamed, roasted or broiled. If possible, avoid all fried foods. Ask for dressings and sauces, to be put on the side. Let's say you're going out with buddies, and you have no choice but to eat fried food and drink tons of beer. Ok, you can compensate by being extra diligent on the days before and after – no late-night eating, no bad snacks.
- Skip breakfast if you eat/drink much the previous night. Intermittent Fasting can be a great help during traveling. Simply wait until 10 a.m. to 12 noon to have your first meal. I usually break my intermittent fast with some lean protein meal, fruit, and some veggies.
- Get creative and think about different ways to exercise at your hotel. Book rooms at a hotel that has a workout facility or a swimming pool. For example, last week I did several circuits walking up and down in the staircases of my hotel.

- Always keep some healthy snacks in your bag – apples, almonds, the small pack of almond butter, protein bars.
- Think quality over quantity. You may not have a lot of time to do a 5-mile run, so just use what you have! When I have less time, my workouts consist of a push exercise (pushups or handstand pushups), a pull exercise (pull ups or chin ups), a leg exercise (lunges or squats), and a core exercise (planks or hanging knee tucks) - all this can be completed in 20 minutes.
- Carry simple and effective exercise tools. I usually carry the following gears in my luggage: a skipping rope, a resistance band, and a Tennis ball. You can use these tools anywhere.

Travel Job: How to avoid or recover from jet lag quickly

Jet lag and flight fatigue is a temporary disorder that causes fatigue, insomnia, and other symptoms as a result of air travel across time zones. It is considered a circadian rhythm sleep disorder, which is a disruption of the internal body clock.

If you are a jet lag sufferer you could also feel anxiety, confusion, headache, difficulty concentrating, etc. This can completely destroy your travel and affect your fitness routine.

Fortunately, jet lag is temporary, and you can recover within a few days if you know what to do.

Here are some tips to quickly recover from jet lag:

- Continue exercising and eating healthy food.
- Avoid using sleeping medication or use it right.
- Go out in sunlight for 15 minutes.
- Walk in a park on grass barefooted.

- During the flight avoid alcohol/caffeine and drink more water.

- Adjust clock sleep as per destination time.

- Drink orange juice.

- Wear comfortable shoes and clothes.

- Walk and exercise.

- Hang upside down. You get blood flow to the head and "decompress" all those sitting and back muscles. I do it for 5 minutes in the morning after a long flight.

The importance of the right breathes in sport

Research carried out by two scientists in 1983 found that runners who breathed in time with their stride had the highest level of performance. More recently, in 2011, a major study at the University of Portsmouth tested 12 runners over a six-week period and discovered that athletes who included breathing exercises as part of their training improved their times by 5-12 percent.

Breathe techniques to improve your sport performance

1. A minute of focus on your breath. Breathe in for a few seconds then exhale for the same amount of time.

2. Diaphragmatic Breathing (AKA deep belly breathing).

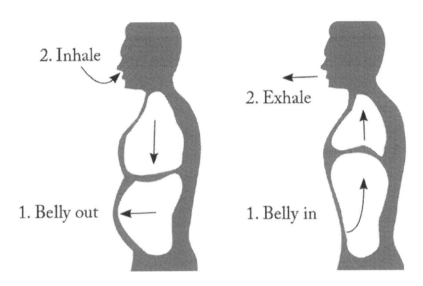

This is a type of breathing when your belly rises and falls with each breath. It is common in babies. This technique activates our parasympathetic nervous system which is our body's rest mechanism. It gives us energy and slows our heart rate. We feel very relaxed, focused, calm and grounded after practicing this. Some other benefits of this practice include improved circulation, calmed nervous system, improved immune system, increased breath capacity.

This is effectively done before training as part of your warm-up or for example ahead of a great event, competition. And also, do it every time you feel stress, anxiety or physical tension in your body.

3. *Long exhale breathing.*

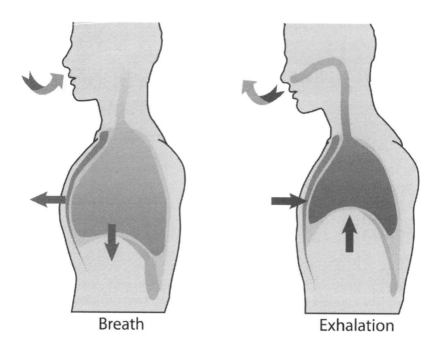

Breath   Exhalation

Here are the steps to do this practice:

- ⬚ Lay in your back, bent your knees, make your feet flat, place one hand on your abdomen, take a few relaxed breaths, lengthen out the inhalation and exhalation to reach the equal length, progressively increase the length of your exhale until you have a 1:2 ratio, continue doing it for 5-10 minutes.

The most important benefit of this technique is that it helps to get good sleep.

How did I doubled my underwater breath hold time in 3 days?

My first baseline hold time was 40 seconds. After practicing the following steps for 3 days I was able to hold my breath under the water for 80 seconds.

1. Practice deep breathing: Start with 60- 90 seconds of "deep breathing". Deep breathing involves taking a deep breath through your mouth, holding for 1 second, then breathing out for 10 seconds with your mouth almost closed.

2. Take out extra Co2 by "Purging". Do a strong long exhalation as if you were trying to blow a toy sailboat across a pool, followed by a big but faster inhalation.

3. Now inhale normally. When you inhale, don't breathe in so much that you're about to pop.

4. Hold your breath for as long as possible. Keep calm and divert your mind.

Fitness for Professionals, Students and Busy People

One thing everyone can agree about living in the modern day is that you're going to have a busy, fast-paced life.

I receive this question all the time:

I'm working 12 hours a day Manjeet, how do I find the time to work out?

Maybe you're too busy with your business, maybe you have 2 hour long commutes and 10 hour workdays, maybe you're a student balancing your part-time job with your classes, maybe you're a busy housewife taking care of 2 kids – we can all agree that life is busy, and there's going to be days where you don't have the time to go to the gym.

Whatever the case, when push comes to shove, people focus on more immediate problems – hustling to make that sale, working your butt off for that promotion, getting your kids ready for school, preparing that client pitch presentation.

Health takes a backseat. This is understandable, but in the long term, deadly. No matter how busy you are, you need to find some time to exercise – the human body was not meant to sit in a chair all day.

You need to figure out how much time you can squeeze out of your day – an hour is great, 45 minutes is good, half an hour is okay, and 15 minutes is the bare minimum. With that said, if you can squeeze just 15 minutes off your day, you can still do quite a bit with it.

Ideally, try to find time in the morning right before you take a bath – this way you can save some time by not having to bathe twice (exercise will leave you sweaty).

Here is the workout I do on busy days:

1. 100 Squats (15 minutes)

2. 60 Pushups (15 minutes)

3. 100 Sit-ups (10 minutes) + 1-minute Plank (3 sets with 1-minute breaks in between sets) (5 minutes) [Totals 15 minutes]

4. A full body stretching routine (15 minutes)

This pretty much covers all essential portions of your body, and if you're doing only this much, you should be fine – you won't be as good as the guy who spends 2 hours in the gym every day, but you'll be leaps and bounds ahead of the average guy. If you can manage only 15 minutes, alternate the above 4 over 4 days. If you can manage 30 minutes, alternate the above over 2 days. (Squats and pushups on one day / sit-ups, planks and stretching on day 2)

Remember, your choices add up over time. When it comes to health, consistency beats randomness

Here are 6 nutrition you need if you are going Vegan

When people ask me for tips on switching to a plant-based diet, they're usually worried about all the things they'll miss out on. "How will I get enough protein?" they ask. But think about it this way: if your vegan diet is rich in whole foods and a variety of fruits and vegetables, you'll actually be getting more of certain nutrients than you were before – like folate from leafy green veg.

However, there are some essential vitamins and minerals that you may be used to getting from meat, dairy and eggs that are harder to come by when you make the plant-based switch. Here are six crucial vitamins and minerals that every vegan – and many vegetarians – need to keep in mind for their health.

1. Vitamin B12
2. Iron
3. Omega-3 Fatty Acids
4. Iodine
5. Vitamin C
6. Calcium

Are healthy habits worth cultivating?

Researchers from the Harvard T.H. Chan School of Public Health looked at data from more than 73,000 women enrolled in the Nurses' Health Study (NHS) who were followed for 34 years, and more than 38,000 men enrolled in the Health Professionals Follow-up Study (HPFS) who were followed for 28 years. These researchers had found that five low-risk lifestyle habits are critical for a longer life expectancy. The more of these habits people had, the longer they lived. The habits were:

A healthy diet, which was calculated and rated based on reports of regularly eating healthy foods like vegetables, fruits, nuts, whole grains, healthy fats, and omega-3 fatty acids, and avoiding less healthy or unhealthy foods like red and processed meats, sugar-sweetened beverages, trans fat, and excess sodium

A **healthy physical activity level**, measured as at least 30 minutes a day of moderate to vigorous activity, like brisk walking

A **healthy body weight**, defined as a normal body mass index (BMI), which is between 18.5 and 24.9

Never smoking, because there is no healthy amount of smoking

Low-risk alcohol intake, measured as between 5 and 15 grams per day for women, and 5 to 30 grams per day for men. Generally, one drink contains about 14 grams of pure alcohol. That's 12 ounces of regular beer, 5 ounces of wine, or 1.5 ounces of distilled spirits.

Even if they had only one of these habits, participants lived two years longer than if they had none. And if by age 50 they regularly practiced all five, women lived an extra 14 years and men lived an extra 12. That's over a decade of extra life!

SECTION 5

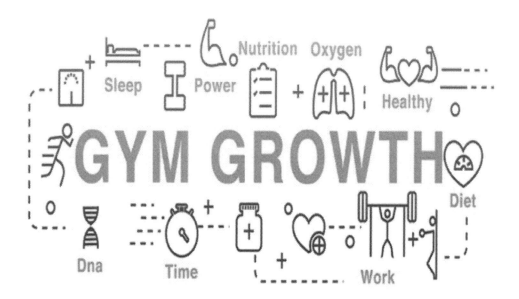

FUTURE OF HEALTH

AND FITNESS

Healthcare & Fitness Integration

You may have been told for many years that the future of the fitness industry is in wellness. But in reality, the future of the industry is really in partnerships with the healthcare community and integrating healthcare and fitness.

While today's healthcare system has intense challenges to sustain long-term, there is a large opportunity for medical leaders and club owners to join forces to redefine healthcare. Medical fitness adoption has yet to reach its potential due to the lack of successful outcomes, integration and profitability.

When I travel around the world I often ask a question where I'm speaking to physician groups "How many of you feel there's an immediate solution to solving the healthcare crisis that we face today?" Not many physicians raise their hand, and it's because a lot of them are frustrated they spend more time in their electronic health records than they do actually give in to give advice.

On the other hand, many fitness professionals are saying hey "we have the time to actually educate to go over nutrition, sleep movement, and corrective exercise to be able to help these patients live a better lifestyle, but there hasn't been a profitable business model". These systems have made in silos and completely separated. For example, there's been medical fitness hospital associations but very little integration communication with fitness professionals.

What we need is a next-level health care model where physicians and fitness professionals integrate together, they communicate together, to where we actually can solve the opioid crisis. We can handle patients and pain management differently. We can truly get to the root cause and really address all these factors through health coaching and personal trainers. Medical professionals that prescribe the treatment plans so there's trust there's communication and back and forth.

ARTIFICIAL INTELLIGENCE AND HEALTHCARE

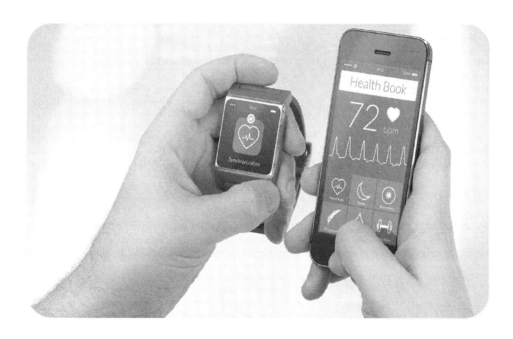

The current system is broken. We need to move towards an era of disease prevention and personalized medicine.

In this age new technologies appear almost every day in every sphere. Health and healthcare aren't an exception. New technologies in healthcare transform people's lives usually for the better. They help people to better track, manage and improve our own health and the health of our family members. We are able to live better in an improved society. With new technologies, healthcare delivery becomes more efficient. Also, healthcare becomes more open, costs are being reduced, quality is increased.

Worldwide, healthcare is at the intersection of ever-rising costs and the introduction of disruptive digital innovations, digital health innovations will expectantly play a significant role in:

- Curbing long-term healthcare costs.
- Enabling better healthcare outcomes.
- Empowering both the patient and the healthcare provider with real-time data and connections with each other.
- Enabling the introduction of new contributors to the healthcare ecosystem.

Imagine a model of healthcare that's always available and driven by data so you're continuously collecting data off your body, about your environment, your nutrition, and activity. Then it delivers back to you personalized health care throughout your whole life. You don't have to be in a brick-and-mortar building to get it, and you have access to the world's best experts.

Our smartphones now are an important part of our lives and in healthcare, they play a major role too. Other important technologies of this field are smart sensors, cloud storage and data analytics.

The most notable benefit of healthcare technologies is that they enable us to early predict the disease and take appropriate actions. It enhances the treatment and leverages the costs. Monitoring technologies give an opportunity to remote monitoring and care of the patients.

The global population is projected to reach 10 billion people by 2050. Chronic diseases are rising: 73% of all deaths are expected to result from chronic diseases by 2020. Populations are aging: the number of people aged 60 years and older will rise from 900 million to 2 billion between 2015 and 2050; that's a rise from 12% to 22% of the total global population. In this new era of digital connection, patients are transitioning from passive healthcare recipients to active value-seeking consumers.

There is enormous potential for digital technology to improve many aspects of health and social care provision. Digital and Mobile Health (mHealth) opportunities have different uses from simple to complicated, from chronic care management to complex population health analysis.

Figure mHealth opportunity uses

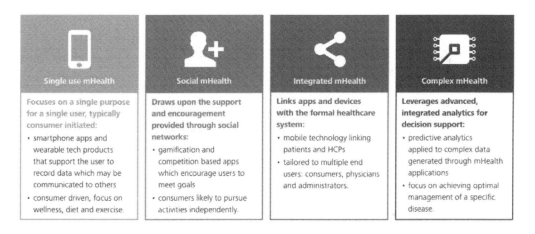

A key development in mHealh is wearable technologies. Most wearable devices transfer data via an app. There are three main characteristics of wearable devices. The functionality and use of increasingly unobtrusive bio-sensing wearables.

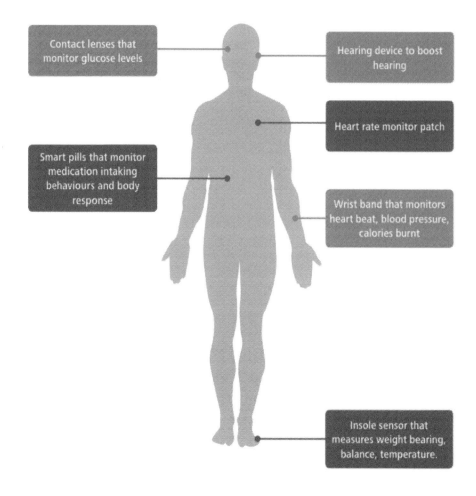

Contact lenses that monitor glucose levels

Hearing device to boost hearing

Heart rate monitor patch

Smart pills that monitor medication intaking behaviours and body response

Wrist band that monitors heart beat, blood pressure, calories burnt

Insole sensor that measures weight bearing, balance, temperature.

Here is a list of best wearable technology devices:

1. **Fitbit Ionic.**

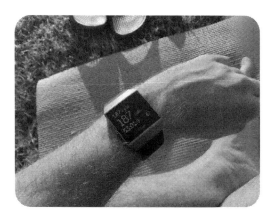

This is Fitbit's strongest smartwatch. This is a dream for every fitness lover. It is able to track whatever workouts you want to manage.

2. **Under Armour Gemini 3 RE smart shoes.**

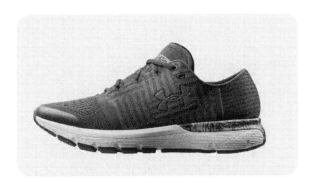

The fitness tracker is right into the soles of the shoes. This is very comfortable because you don't need to wear smartwatches which are easy to drop, break or lose. The shoes record running metrics and have Bluetooth connectivity to connect with the app.

3. Spire and Swim.com smart swimsuits.

This device tracks your pool time and automatically sends the data to the swim.com app.

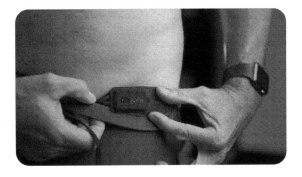

4. Myontec Mbody connected shorts.

The special bit of skit claims to offer "the most comprehensive and advanced training system available" with its Mbody fitness-tracking hip-huggers. Mbody is designed especially for cyclists, duathletes, and triathletes by collecting combined muscle load with heart rate data, such as cadence, speed and distance, via its MCell Smart measuring tech. This technology measures the electrical activity of the muscles (EMG, electromyography) and is apparently the first of its kind to do so in real-time sports performance analysis, regardless of the environment or the type of sport.

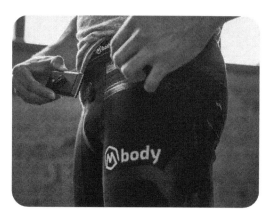

5.Coros smart bicycle helmet

This bicycle helmet has bone-conduction earphones built in which gives you an opportunity to safely listen to music or GPS directions while you ride the streets. Moreover, it tracks your mileage and will send an automatic and immediate message to your relative in case of any accident. And, of course, it is very beautiful and looks smart.

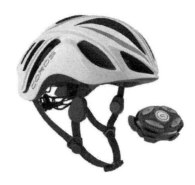

There are many other devices with different features and prices. You can research for them and choose the one that will be helpful for your fitness needs.

3D PRINTING

On-demand manufacturing will make medical devices cheaper and more readily accessible to millions, and it will make scarce resources like organs-for-transplant abundantly available.

3D Systems is 3D printing precise dental and anatomical models, custom surgical guides, implantable devices, exoskeletons, hearing aids, prosthetics and braces for scoliosis and other applications.

Students at Washington University 3D printed a robotic arm for about $200. Traditional robotic limbs can run $50,000 to $70,000, and they need to be replaced as children grow. Companies like Organovo are 3D bio-printing with cells to produce tissues, blood vessels and even small organs.

Genomics & Big Data

The cost of genome sequencing has plummeted 100,000-fold, from $100M per genome in 2001 to $1,000 per genome today... outpacing Moore's Law by 3x.

Once companies have a large amount of gnome data, they would be able to unlock the secrets of our biology. We'll find insights into and cures for cancer, heart disease and neurodegenerative disease, and ultimately extend the human lifespan.

Stem Cells

We are now in the earliest stages of stem cell therapy development. Future therapies will be transformative and, frankly, mind-boggling.

Stem cell therapy promises tissue regeneration and renewal – and thus a "cure" for everything from blindness to spinal cord injuries, Type 1 diabetes, Parkinson's disease, Alzheimer's disease, heart disease, stroke, burns, cancer and osteoarthritis.

In 2012, researchers at Cedars-Sinai reported one of the first cases of successful therapeutic stem cell treatment – they used patients' own stem cells to regenerate heart tissue and undo damage from a heart attack.

FUTURE OF FITNESS

The technology driving fitness now breaks down into three categories: performance improvement, experiencing the gym in new ways and marketplaces.

Working out at home is now a trend.

It is a seasonal fad that peaks in the winter months when people have made New Year's resolutions and home workouts are not likely to grow overall. There are a few companies that have grown rapidly in the home workout market and they are rare exceptions. Most notable is Peloton but most other equipment makers are targeted at clubs or have not been nearly as successful as Peloton in reaching consumers buying home workout equipment.

Community in gym workouts is the top motivator for consumers to go to gyms.

The data are not clear whether the social motivator for going to gyms is the obligation to a trainer or class or whether the social interactions consumers have with fellow members is the catalyst or whether it's just having other people around. But social experiences at gyms is by far the highest motivating factor for joining and going. Having a professional setup in a gym is also rated highly.

Technology development in fitness is growing and consumers are driving that growth.

Although technology is not spurring more interest in home workouts, fitness apps are widely used at gyms and in outdoor workout and fitness settings. Fitbit is the best known of such devices; interest in that specific product has peaked. (Google has agreed to buy Fitbit, no doubt to leverage the health information it has gathered. With revenues and earnings off its peak, the deal could be a good way to reinvigorate the brand.)

Coaching and Performance Improvement

Fitness companies are using new technology to help amateurs be better at their sport with real-time, personalized instruction that uses artificial intelligence (AI). An AI program created by a company called Asensei which puts sensors in your workout clothes to monitor your movements. It can then give you highly specific instructions about how to move your body based on what it senses through your clothing. At the moment, it works for yoga and rowing. Companies are now working with apparel manufacturers to incorporate its technology into branded garments.

Moving the Gym to New Venues

Companies are changing the way gyms are experienced. A user in a gym puts on a virtual reality headset and attaches to weights made for the purpose. A video game begins in which there's no hand-held controller, the user's body movements control the game. As the user moves, the weights are lifted. Because of the weights a user gets a complete workout by the time a game is over. If you love playing video games but are not highly motivated to work out in a gym, this will bring you in and keep you there. Like other video games, it is always changing and evolving based on your skill. It is designed to be played either against the computer or against other people who can be either nearby or anywhere else in the world.

Another company called Forte moves the gym class to any other location in the world. It installs hardware and software into workout studios and gyms to bring live and on-demand fitness classes to consumers when they can't make classes at the gym. Interestingly, Forte has found that consumers prefer live classes because they are real and authentic over recorded or repeated content.

Marketplaces

Like so many other sectors, gyms and fitness are seeing the development of marketplaces that match providers with users. One of those is Athlete's Guide, a digital marketplace that connects NCAA athletes with high school athletes to help them train better and mentor the younger athletes. The appeal of the experience is for high school athletes to work with a role model in something that the younger students are highly engaged with. Parents of high school students like it as a way to enhance their child's skill as well as keep them involved with sports.

Fittr is a community-based health & fitness app with everything you need to start your transformation journey; It's like having your own fitness coach with a huge community supporting you wherever you go!

Here is my prediction on 10 meta trends in 2020s that will significantly improve how the fitness and healthcare work today.

1. Global gigabit connectivity will connect everyone and everything, everywhere, at an ultra-low cost
2. Continued increase in global abundance - decrease in poverty
3. The average human health span will increase by 10+ years
4. AI-Human Collaboration will skyrocket across all professions
5. Autonomous vehicles and flying cars will redefine human travel
6. On-demand production and on-demand delivery will birth an "instant economy of things.
7. Ability to sense and know anything, anytime, anywhere Increased focus on sustainability and the environment
8. CRISPR and gene therapies will minimize disease
9. Everything is smart, embedded with intelligence
10. Globally abundant, cheap renewable energy

Do I still have a need for a Personal Trainer?

People buy trainers - not training.

How can a great trainer help?

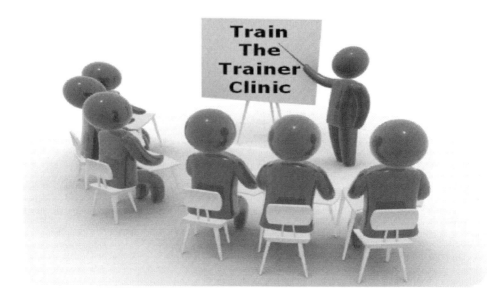

People hate to be sold but love to buy. Once I have moved into personal training, I have realized that a job of a great trainer is not to just create workout plans and sold sessions– but to focus on client needs, value, emotions and always strive to meet the clients at their level.

When people ask me to provide a workout or diet plan, my usual response is: "you can find a reasonably good plan by a simple google search or buy a $5 fitness magazine. You do not need a trainer if you are just looking for a workout/fitness nutrition plan.

The best coaches are not the ones who know how to give advice but the ones who brings following things to table:

Accountability. So many of us make New Year fitness goals and then derail from the plan within a few weeks. A great trainer should be able to keep you on track no matter what.

Emotion. A trainer should be able to build trust so that clients can open up and talk about their emotions, needs and feelings more freely. Many trainers push their programs on new clients without asking themselves if those programs fulfil the client's wants and needs. Your trainers must think of members first, not their own programs.

Supporter. There are days when clients might be in a bad state when they come into the gym. If I sense that something is wrong with my client, I'd ask them to talk to me about it before we start the session.

Find Common ground. Clients invest in your products or services because they have problems or needs that you can help them fix. Your trainers must become experts at understanding members' specific situations and at uncovering their pressing needs. Your trainers must show members how training can change their lives and solve their emotional pain and follow through with their promises of help.

Expectation. Our world thrives on looking young and beautiful. So even though many clients desire to be healthy and to increase their longevity, the underlying truth is that everyone wants to look good. Your trainers should help paint a "before and after" picture with some reasonable expectations around how much time, dedication and hard work would need to reach to that level.

Passion. Trainers with enthusiasm and passion transmit that energy to their clients.

Friendship. A great trainer always strives to build a friendship, be approachable and ready to help even after the program has ended.

What are the advantages of a personal trainer over group exercise?

The most important benefit of having a trainer is reduced risk of injury. While boot camps and Cross Fit are motivating to some folks, the instructor to athlete ratio is so low that improper form goes unnoticed or is simply ignored. Joint pain and injury inevitably surface when poor form isn't addressed.

I already work out, what would I gain from a formal exercise program?

The result will be your best body. Every gym-goer gets stuck in a routine at some point and plateaus. Push Fitness personalized fitness programs are rooted in progressions. Continually advancing some aspect of your fitness level is the difference between training and exercise and therefore the difference between results and plateaus.

How frequently should I see a trainer?

The ideal frequency of personal training sessions varies from person to person. Just getting started with exercise and healthy eating? Need regular motivation and support to get to the gym? Have an injury that you're working through? You'll probably need to see a trainer once or twice each week. Many of my weekly clients reduce their frequency of personal training sessions to bi-weekly or even monthly once they've demonstrated the ability to consistently get to the gym and progress their exercises as recommended.

Although I miss seeing their smiling faces, I'm always pleased when clients reduce their need to see me because they've become self-directed exercise.

As we use more digital devices and other equipment, we will create more waste on the earth. We all should be collectively responsible for keeping this earth clean, water clean and air clean.

Five Eco Hacks to Help Planet and Reduce Waste

From the cars we drive to the food we eat, elements of our everyday life are contributing to global CO_2 emissions and polluting our air and waterways.

You don't have to turn full eco-warrior, but if we all implement a few tiny changes to our everyday lives, we'll help the environment and get a whole lot of benefits on the side and contribute in reducing increase risk of global warming.

1. Reduce your waste.

 Did you hear about the woman who can fit two years of trash into one small mason jar? It's extreme, but doable. Looking at ways to reduce your waste will significantly help the Earth, and might save you money, too.

A good place to start is with your produce shopping. You'll find that buying direct from your local fruit and veg store or farmers market usually comes with a lot of less unnecessary packaging and plastic than the big chain supermarkets.

Soft plastic recycling (such as the bag your pasta comes in, or the wrapping around paper towel) is also becoming more common, so look out for schemes in your area.

And we've all been guilty of buying too much, then letting it go off in the bottom of the fridge. Plan in advance and only buy what you need.

2. Create a compost.

Food scraps like fruit and vegetable skins are the perfect inclusion for a compost bin. You can also throw in tea bags and plant cuttings. This will decompose back into the earth and enrich our soils, rather than clogging landfill.

3. Keep your cup.

Reusable coffee cups are now everywhere. While billions of non-degradable coffee cups are being poured into landfill each year, the increasing popularity of reusable coffee cups, with brands like Keep Cup taking off around the world, is a positive sign.

4. Eat less meat.

The Guardian reports that avoiding meat and dairy is the single biggest way you can reduce your carbon footprint. Research shows that producing beef results in up to 105 kg (231 lbs.) of greenhouse gases per 100g (3.5 oz) of meat. Meanwhile, tofu produces less than 3.5 kg (7.7 lbs.). Even the occasional substitution of a vegetarian or vegan dish into your meal plan will have a positive impact.

5. Hop on your bike.

Cars emit huge amounts of greenhouse gas. Walking or riding a bike to work every day (or even a couple of days a week) will save you money and contribute to saving the environment. Plus, think of all those extra calories you'll burn. Win-win.

Conclusion and Summary

This book is written as a daily reference. This book captures the practice philosophies, tactics that has worked for and my clients. So even if you read it through cover to cover, keep it with you. Our memories are flawed. So, whenever you feel that you are going out of track – open this book and there is a high chance that it will bring you to the track.

If you are tired or bored, just remember that you can handle it. Life is about resilience and keep going.

Quotes I live by everyday:
- Agile Fitness Daily practice – become 1% better every day and change the world.
- A fit body, a calm mind, a house full of love. These things cannot be bought - they must be earned.
- You do not rise to the level of your goals. You fall to the level of your systems.
- You should be far more concerned with your current trajectory than with your current results

Read more, use logic and question everything that's happening. That's the only way you'll benefit your body as well as people around you.

I hope this small book gave you enough information to start with. Feel free to share it among your friends and family as well.

Remember, Fitness is your right, but you have to earn it! If you quit now...you will end up where you first began. And when you first began, you were desperate to be right where you are now. Keep going!

References

1. Gretchen, et al. Menstrual cycle phase and oral contraceptive effects on triglyceride mobilization during exercise. J ApplPhysiol 2004;97: 302â€"309.

2. D'eon et al. The Roles of Estrogen and Progesterone in Regulating Carbohydrate and Fat Utilization at Rest and during Exercise. Journal women's health and gender-based medicine 2002;11(3):225-237.

3. Nakamura et al. Hormonal Responses to Resistance Exercise during Different Menstrual Cycle States. Medicine & Science in Sports & Exercise. 2011 Jun;43(6):967-73

4. Oosthuyse& Bosch. The Effect of the Menstrual Cycle on Exercise Metabolism. Sports Medicine. 2010;4(3):207-227.

5. Davis, et al. concurrent training enhances athletes' strength, muscle endurance, and other measures. Journal of Strength and Conditioning Research. 2008 September;22(5):1487-1502.

6. National Strength & Conditioning Association. Essentials of strength training & conditioning. Champaign, IL: Human Kinetics. 2000

7. stronglifts.com/5-reasons-why-you-shouldnt-do-static-stretches/

8. http://www.womenshealthmag.com/fitness/period-workout

9. http://www.bodybuilding.com/fun/sclark109.htm

10. http://www.runnersworld.com/

11. http://www.bengreenfieldfitness.com and https://lifemathmoney.com/

Made in the USA
Las Vegas, NV
22 April 2022

47834150R00118